I DARED TO DREAM

My Journey with Cochlear Implants

Julie Husting

I Dared to Dream
Copyright © 2020 by Julie Husting

blog: https://juliehusting.wordpress.com/
ISBN: 978-1-71699-751-8

To my brother, Steve,

For taking this journey with me

Preface

This book originally began as a series of emails that I sent to my loved ones when I first received my cochlear implant. A friend suggested that I should write a blog instead, as others might be able to benefit from my experiences. I thought she was crazy, but I did it anyway. The content of this book comes directly from my blog: juliehusting.wordpress.com.

This book spans the first six years of my life with cochlear implants and is written in chronological order. For the continuation of my journey beyond the scope of this book, as well as the pictures that go along with these stories, be sure to visit my blog.

This book is simply my story. I am not a medical professional. Any information, advice and recommendations are based purely on my own experiences and beliefs. Each person's level of success with a cochlear implant varies and is dependent on many factors. The content of this book is not intended to be a substitute for professional medical advice, diagnosis, or treatment. Always seek the advice of your physician or other qualified health provider with any questions you have regarding a medical condition.

I hope that this book inspires others to consider a cochlear implant just as Arlene Romoff's book, *Listening Closely: A Journey to Bilateral Hearing* inspired me to get my second cochlear implant. As a mentor, I come in contact with people just beginning this journey on a regular basis. I can relate to their experiences and I am happy to be a part of their journeys. I know what a miracle is waiting for them but I also know what fear of the unknown feels like. If my story can turn one person's fear into excitement then it will all be worthwhile.

Go ahead . . . Dare to Dream!

My early years

I had perfect hearing up until I was seventeen. My brother, Steve, was five when he began losing his hearing. I have only known him as a person with a hearing loss. As far as I can remember, his hearing was always really poor.

All through my school years I enjoyed public speaking, debates, and theater. I was also usually ahead of the other kids in my classes and numerous teachers over the years would have me tutor the kids that were behind. It was really gratifying helping those kids because I could see them doing better in school. I really enjoyed doing that. I had decided that, when I grew up, I wanted to be a lawyer or a fourth-grade teacher.

Then one day I was sitting at the table reading a book and my mom was trying to talk to me. I kept reading my book and she grew madder and madder because I was ignoring her. I had no idea she was talking to me. She thought I was just being a rebellious teenager. That's the day we knew something was wrong with my hearing.

She immediately got me an appointment in Los Angeles with one of the best hearing specialists around. He said that my hearing loss was hereditary, and that there was no surgery that could correct the problem. I remember the appointment when I got my hearing aids very clearly. We were in a high rise building and I heard some kind of loud noise but had no idea what it was. It was a garbage truck on the street below. I also kept hearing a swishing sound and nobody could figure out what that was. That turned out to be my hair rubbing on my nylon jacket every time I turned my head.

I had gotten a job when I was sixteen photocopying reports and doing mailings for a financial investment firm. I was promoted to secretary and transcribed the reports that my boss wrote. I know I had to hear to do that and I did it well.

I got married when I was nineteen, worked full time during the day, and went to college at night. I was always a straight "A" student all the way through high school but college was another matter. I still did fairly well but it was a struggle to hear and it didn't help that the majority of the professors had foreign accents. I worked full time during the day and went to school at night for ten years. It was only in the last year that I found out that I could have someone take notes for me. The college offered that service to hearing impaired students. I did take them up on that and it was easier, but how I wish I had known that earlier.

I had long ago given up my dream of becoming a lawyer or a teacher. Lawyers have to be able to hear well in a courtroom, and it's necessary to be able to hear to be a fourth grade teacher. Children with high voices were especially hard for me to understand. Fortunately, I had always liked using calculators and was very good with money so I decided to become an accountant instead. I've had a long career in accounting and have done quite well for myself, but I still have a dream of teaching. It's always been just a dream but now, with this implant, maybe it can become a reality someday. If it's not in a classroom, then possibly tutoring again.

Dreams are usually just that for a person with a disability. A guy in a wheelchair can only dream of running a marathon, for example. It's just not going to happen. I had the choice to feel sorry for myself for the things that I couldn't do or I could concentrate on what I could do and have a good, fulfilling life. Oh sure, every now and then I would throw a pity party for myself but there really wasn't any point in that. I simply accepted my limitations and moved on. It could have been a pretty miserable life if I hadn't!

JULIE HUSTING

Deciding to Get a Cochlear Implant

I've lived my life and had adapted to my "moderate" hearing loss. A few years ago I purchased new top of the line hearing aids. It turns out I hated them. Oh sure, they were loud enough but they were far too noisy in social settings. By this time, I was relying quite heavily on reading lips. It's not something I was conscious of doing but as soon as someone looked away, covered their mouth, or it was dark and I couldn't see their lips, I realized I was doing it.

When I went to the audiologist to get new hearing aids a few months ago I was shocked when she told me I had a "profound" hearing loss and was asked if I had considered getting a cochlear implant. Wait! What? How could that be? That's Steve she's talking about, not me! I have a "moderate" hearing loss. Steve's the one that's deaf! But I looked at the hearing test and saw that the lines were all the way down at the bottom of the chart. That was quite a wakeup call.

I began to think about all of the things I have been missing. Remember, I have not been one to dwell on those things. I've dealt with it and moved on. But I stopped to really think about it. It is especially difficult to understand in noisy situations. Notice I didn't say "hear." I said "understand." What hearing people don't understand about hearing aids is that they are plenty loud enough (sometimes too loud) they just aren't clear. They served me well most of my life but I began to think about all of the times that I couldn't understand: restaurants, rubber stamping (my hobby) with other people, in groups of people, in cars, etc. Because I have to read lips, I can't look down and stamp and listen to the conversations around me at the same time. I know I've missed out on a lot of juicy details of my stamping friends' lives.

I went home and read a little bit about cochlear implants. I knew about them before but thought that they were permanent, ie that you'd hear 24/7. That didn't appeal to me. I *like* not being able to hear when I go to bed. My partner, Bob's, snoring is horrendous and I don't have to listen to that. I also don't hear rain, thunder, lawnmowers, TV's blaring, etc. It's peaceful, and I usually get a good night's sleep. I also thought I'd have this big thing sticking out of my head that everybody would see and that I'd have to wear this big thing around my neck. I also thought it would cost $100,000.

Cochlear implants would be great for someone like Steve. I asked him why he hadn't gotten one. He said he didn't want to spend the money. I understood, but it was a shame because a cochlear implant could change his life.

I went back to my audiologist to pick up the hearing aids. I mentioned the implants to her and told her that they were too expensive. She then told me something that would change my life forever. She said insurance pays 100% for them. She then gave me the number of Debbie and Al in Huntington Beach. Al had gotten an implant about a year ago, and he lived just a few miles away from me.

I called Steve right away, and then I called Al. Steve and his wife, Shirley, and I went and met with Al and Debbie. Before talking to Al and Debbie, I had already decided that Steve should be the guinea pig. He could get the implant first and then, if he could actually hear better than I could, I would get one. But then we met Al and Debbie. That one hour conversation did it. I was in total amazement talking to them. He didn't have some strange thing protruding from his head. Yes, he was wearing something but it was about the size of a quarter and looked like a button. He didn't have to wear a big old thing around his neck either. I guess implants had changed quite a bit from when I had first heard of them. To my surprise, he could now do everything that I couldn't. His wife was also very happy. It's been so much easier for her.

Steve and I were both convinced. We had to get a cochlear implant! Rather than waiting for Steve to get his, it was now a race to see who could get theirs first. We were both very excited and full of hope after leaving there. We both got the ball rolling with our respective doctors the next day.

From Testing to Surgery

Steve had his CT scan done and I had the first hearing test. Then he had his first hearing test and I had my second. Then I got my CT scan done and

Steve, unfortunately, had a hiccup with his doctor. They didn't submit the paperwork for him to move forward. He's been stalled for a couple of months.

In the meantime, I met with the surgeon, Dr. Shohet, who suggested that I have both ears implanted. The first ear would be implanted now and the second ear would be done three to six months later. I immediately said no and I told him why. I am convinced that technology will drastically change in the rest of my lifetime. I was worried that I would not be able to take advantage of new technology if I ruin my ears now. When they do the surgery they damage part of the ear and there is no residual hearing left which means that things like hearing aids will never work on the ear again, nor will you be able to take advantage of future technology that might require an intact ear. I was also concerned that cochlear technology is only about twenty-five years old. What if it the internal implant shorts out in twenty years? Once you have the surgery, you are completely deaf. I did not want to wind up completely deaf in twenty years.

He told me that the longer I wait, the more my auditory nerve will deteriorate. The better the nerve, the better I would do with the implant. He also said that the major technological changes are made to the outside processors, not the internal implant. I have to wear a processor that is, basically, a mini computer that talks to the implant that's imbedded in my head. Whenever they come up with new advances they update the software in the processor. Sometimes they come out with new processors altogether, but they still "talk" to the implant in my head. I can rest assured that whatever new advances they come up with in the next ten years (and likely much longer) I will be able to take advantage of.

I told him I had heard about stem cell research that they are doing now and he stated that it would not be ready for a good ten to twenty years at the earliest. After that, who knows what the future holds for hearing? I still was not convinced and I told the audiologist my concerns. She said that they would be testing the hearing aid ear every year and as soon as she noticed a change, we could talk about getting the implant then. That sounded like a good plan to me. Many people, including Al, wear the implant in one ear and a hearing aid in the other ear. This is called "bimodal."

Well, all of that discussion was *before* the implant was turned on. Now, of course, I can see for myself how great it is. I'm convinced that, if I continue to improve the way I think I will, I will be perfectly happy with what I am hearing, now, for the rest of my life and I don't care what the future holds. Yes, the wires on the Neptune processor will likely become archaic but I can live with that. I would rather hear well in both ears, now, than live with a bad ear for another ten to twenty years hoping that there will be something better. What if there's not? Then I wasted a lot of time. Al, by the way, is working on getting his second implant now.

I have to mention what the tests were like that I took. In order to be approved for an implant you have to have a "severe to profound" hearing loss. They do very detailed tests. There is the standard "beep" test that you take when getting hearing aids. Then they do a word list with the hearing aids on. They said fifty words. Since I couldn't read lips I only got two words right, which is just 4%. Not good. Then they did a sentence test. They had a recording that played a ton of sentences. I had to say any word that I could understand. I didn't answer any of those. I failed those tests miserably, which in actuality, meant I passed. So far so good.

I went back for more tests. The next tests were to test me for balance and vertigo. I had to stare at a big screen TV while checkerboards flew past, and try not to watch them, but focus straight ahead. Easier said than done! Then came what I call "the New Year's Eve at my brother, Curtis', party test." I laid down on a table and then they put black goggles on me that I couldn't see through. Those measured my eye movement. Then they turned out the lights and shot a stream of cold air through my ear. Whoa! I felt like I had ten kamikazes, and a few margaritas to boot. My eyeballs swooshed all over the place. Then she turned it off and had me start counting by fours. At this point I was supposed to keep my eyes straight ahead. If you've ever been drunk and then laid down, you know that the room is spinning around and this was no different. Wow! Then she did the test again on the other ear, then twice more using hot air. I had the same results. Cheapest buzz I've ever had. Surprisingly, she told me I passed the test.

I then had to make the big decision of choosing which implant I wanted. I did a lot of research. I knew I wanted to go with the company that had the best technology. I also knew that technology changes, and I wanted a company that would keep improving. I wanted to be able to take advantage of the changes in technology over the years. I found the website, Cochlear Implant

Help (cochlearimplanthelp.com). It has a great side-by-side comparison chart on all three of the companies that produce cochlear implants. Since technology was the most important factor in determining which implant I chose, I took the information to an engineer friend of mine and asked for his opinion. He said he would go with Advanced Bionics. I have since learned more about virtual channels, how electrodes work, and input dynamic range (IDR). I discuss some of these topics later in this book. My friend gave me good advice.

Next came the waiting for the insurance approval. That seemed to take forever. I knew I was going to have to have the three P's once I got the implant: patience, practice, and persistence. I guess maybe this was a test of my patience. Finally, I got a surgery date of October 18, 2012.

Advanced Bionics has a fantastic website. They have a forum where you can ask questions and people who have implants will answer with their experience. It's called Hearing Journey (www.HearingJourney.com). You can also read past posts. It's been a great help to me and I was lucky that I knew what to expect ahead of time.

For the surgery, I was told that I would likely get pretty sick afterwards and might have a problem with dizziness for a few days. Fortunately, none of that happened to me. I didn't even need pain medication. I just took Tylenol on occasion. I did have loss of taste on some foods. They tasted very bland for about six months. My mouth was a bit dry, too. I also heard strange creaking sounds in my head from time to time, and my tinnitus would roar like a burst from a fog horn for brief moments. Fortunately, those sounds ended once I was activated. I was off of work for a week. I was very tired and had to force myself to just relax and stay on the couch. The first couple of nights I slept on my recliner. It helps to have your head elevated in the beginning. Some people use neck pillows like you wear on an airplane. I had to wait about three weeks after the surgery until the big day — activation!

During the three week wait, I dared to dream. It's a whole different ballgame dreaming when you know that those dreams might actually come true! I wore the hearing aid in my left ear, and during that time I thought about everything that I couldn't hear and made up a "hearing wish list." These are the things that I am hoping one day to be able to hear. Surprisingly I've already crossed some of the items off.

Here's the list so far:

- Understand at plays / musicals / concerts
- Understand what characters and voiceovers are saying on rides at amusement parks
- Understand what my fellow stamping friends are saying when we are stamping
- Understand what my customers are saying when they come over for Stamp Night and are chatting with each other
- Understand what speakers at seminars and meetings are saying
- Understand what my geocaching friends are saying when we meet up and it's dark outside
- Understand what people are saying in the car
- Hearing birds
- Be able to tell when bikes are coming up behind me when I'm hiking
- Understand what is being said at the movies
- Tinnitus gone or lessened
- Hearing my cat purr
- Understand in restaurants easily
- Understand a whole joke from start to finish
- Understand on the phone without assistance

November 6, 2012 Activation Day

As you know, I had my surgery on October 18, 2012. Today was the day they turned the electrodes on. Wow! What a day it's been so far. Here's a little background, in case you don't know. The surgery put the implant in the cochlear in my ear. The implant has sixteen electrodes that stimulate the auditory nerve. Since I have the Advanced Bionics implant, the electrodes have independent power sources and have 120 virtual channels. It's a completely different way of hearing than what I have been hearing for most of my life with the hearing aids. Because of this, the brain has to relearn how to hear all over again.

Fortunately, from reading Hearing Journey, I was very prepared when I went in today to expect the worst and hope for the best. Many people cannot understand anything at all when they are first activated. Some people hear Darth Vader voices, some hear Mickey Mouse, and some hear more robotic voices. Many people can't make out speech at all. I expected, and was emotionally prepared, to not understand speech at all.

I went in and saw the surgeon first. He checked me over and said I was completely healed and could resume all activities. Then I went to see the audiologist, Cheryl, for the activation. My parents came with me.

The internal implant is one part. The other part is the external processor. I got the Advanced Bionics Neptune processor. That consists of a head piece that has a magnet that sticks to my head which is sticking to the internal part that's under my skin. The head piece has a cord that attaches to the processor. The processor has a triple A battery and the computer programs.

While Cheryl was putting the processor together, I explained to Dad what was happening. Cheryl was pretty impressed by how much I knew. That's all thanks to the forum. Then she turned the electrodes on. This part of the process was supposed to be a series of beeps and I was supposed to tell her when it got to the "comfortable" part. Well, that's pretty difficult to do. For one thing, it's listening to annoying beeps and annoying beeps aren't comfortable. I think we both got a little frustrated so she just went ahead and turned it all on at once. Then I could hear her voice and she could figure out the volume that way.

I cracked up when I heard her voice. She sounded like she was on helium. I could understand everything she was saying. I was reading her lips but it was all clear, just extremely funny. She had Mom and Dad talk, and Dad sounded like a five year old girl. I really laughed when I heard that. Mom sounded like Cheryl on helium, too. We laughed quite a bit and then Cheryl had me close my eyes and she told me the days of the week and had me repeat them back to her, at least what I heard anyway. I'm not sure how many of those I got right but I was amazed that I understood her at all with my eyes closed. That's not easy to do with hearing aids. I very much rely on lipreading.

She did more adjustments and then I just cried. I was so prepared not to understand any speech and was so overwhelmed by it all that I just couldn't help myself. I'm pretty sure I couldn't stop smiling. Actually, I'm not sure I've stopped yet.

We were probably there almost a couple of hours and then we went back to Mom and Dad's house. When I got out of the car, I heard this strange noise. I looked around it was a guy that had a big broom who was sweeping water in the street. Wow! I couldn't believe I could hear that.

I had typed up "closed" lists of words as a rehab exercise. They were made up of colors, holidays, months, days of the week, family names, and animals. I had Dad read the lists to me while I had my back to him and I repeated the words back to him. He checked off the ones I got right. About halfway through I just started crying. Poor Dad. He thought I was upset because I missed a couple, but in reality, I was crying because I could hear him so clearly and I was getting so many words right. I wasn't expecting to be able to do that today. It is a miracle!

Then I took the list in to Mom and she did the same thing, but she mixed up the order of the words. Some of the words that I couldn't understand when Dad said them, I got right when she said them. I got most of the words right again. Keep in mind I had not worn the hearing aid in my other ear since I was at the doctor's office. This was all only using the implant. My left ear, the un-implanted side, only hears ringing from tinnitus.

Mom then decided to get fancy on me and tried "open" sets of words. Those are just random words that I have no idea what they should be. I didn't do very well at that. That's pretty advanced.

We went to lunch at a tiny restaurant, and that was a whole new adventure. When we drove to the restaurant I heard another noise periodically that I didn't recognize. It turns out it was when the asphalt changed from smooth to a little different type of asphalt. The restaurant chairs were *horrible*. They were very loud when we pulled our chairs out and pushed them in. Every now and then I heard this really loud noise and Mom said it was the waitress putting ice in the cups and filling up the drinks. There were more chipmunks/helium sounding people in the restaurant but I couldn't understand what they were saying. There was also a noise that sounded like rain throughout the whole time we were there. I never did figure out what that was.

Then we went to the library. It's good therapy for me to listen to audiobooks and read along with the written book. I heard that it's good to try simple books to start, so I chose a book that I remembered from my childhood. I'll get a kick out of reading that one again. I selected a couple of Dean Koontz books, too.

Then we went back to Mom's. On the way to the library, Dad was sitting in the back seat and I was sitting directly in front of him in the front seat. I had Dad read various signs that we passed that we both could see. Then I repeated them back to him. I could understand all of them. "Wienerschnitzel" was the word that left me in hysterics today. It was just too funny listening to my dad, the five-year-old girl, say that word. I made him say it a couple of times. By the way, this was something else that was truly incredible to me. Normally, if I am sitting in the front seat or anywhere in the car for that matter, I have to read a person's lips in order to understand what they are saying. So for me to know which signs Dad was reading, and there were a lot that he didn't read, was a pretty big deal. I wasn't reading his lips. I was just listening.

On the way home, I put Styx' Greatest Hits on my car radio. I know those songs by heart. I wasn't expecting to even know which songs were playing. I have a hard time in the car understanding any of the music with my hearing aids. I have heard that people with implants have a very difficult time with music at first. To my surprise, I knew which songs were playing. I could hear the music, although it all sounded very strange, and I could hear the melody. I couldn't understand the words, but I could hear the voices and I could sing along. Of course, they were on helium, too.

A couple things sounded normal today: the fountains at the library, and my feet on the plastic protector mat on the floor in front of Dad's computer.

All in all, I'm ecstatic! I go to the office tomorrow and I have a feeling it's really going to be a funny day listening to all of my co-workers on helium.

I have a very long road ahead of me. I have a lot of homework to do to get to where I want to be. Fortunately, I've joined an email group that sends out listening exercises every day and we report back what we've heard.

I'm very grateful that cochlear implant technology is available and that I was able to have the surgery while I still have half of my life to live to take advantage of it. I'm also grateful that my parents are alive to witness this miracle and go through this journey with me.

November 13, 2012 # Week One with the New Implant

I've been activated a little over a week now. I thought I'd give a little report on what a great week it's been! I think I might be able to cross off one of my hearing wish list items very soon.

Sounds I have heard this week:

- Bob's cellphone ringing in the house
- washer — including water going in and the spin cycle — from a different room
- a siren from far away while I was outside
- leaves crunching under my feet (I loved this one so much I sought out more leaves and stomped all over them!)
- wind
- gardener trimming the hedges outside my office window
- door opening and closing
- copy machine in the bullpen area outside my office door
- giant staple machine in shipping department at work
- co-worker's heels clacking on the floor
- brother's feet dragging on the floor

Progress I have made: On day one, when I had my dad read the signs when we were driving in the car, I could only understand the words that I could see. The same was true when my co-workers read signs to me. Yesterday, it was too easy so I had my co-worker give me random words instead. It turns out I could understand *everything* she was saying behind me in the car — not just the words she was giving me but the things she was saying to the driver or under her breath, too. I had her sit in the front seat on the way back to work and I could understand most of what she said there, too. That was on my wish list. Now I want to try a car with more people in it and see if I can understand easily or not.

On day one, I put in a seminar CD for background sounds to listen to. I heard, "blah blah blah demonstrator blah blah blah". On Tuesday, I put in an audiobook on chapters that I had already read as background noise. I understood a *lot* of words and knew right where they were on the story. Big words, too.

On day one, all voices were on helium, especially women. Yesterday, my female co-worker almost sounded like her old self. Most men have lower voices now, and are very close to their old voices. Bob sounds the same as he used to and so do my brothers and Dad. Most women are still high and some men are, too.

Last week, if I yelled out to my co-worker on the other side of the wall I couldn't understand her response. Now I can and, not only that, I can hear her talking on the phone and can even make out a word now and then.

On day one, I had to read along with the ESL rehab exercise conversations in order to understand them. When I had my hearing aid (HA) I couldn't understand anything either. Now I can understand it without looking at the words.

Things that remain difficult: noise in restaurants, whistling sounds I hear in music (not real whistling but that's what it sounds like), and car noise. I *can* hear instruments well though. Guitars, drums and violins all sound perfect. Vocals are funny because they are not their voices yet but, if I know the CD, I know which songs are playing and I know what words they are on. Sometimes I can understand some words clearly if it's a song I don't know and I can understand the words on the songs I do know. I'm sure it's because I know those words. I can follow along on the entire song. I couldn't do that in the car with my HAs before. It was difficult to even know which song they were on in the car.

I haven't worn my other HA and I am pretty much deaf in that ear. There is no sound without the HA on. I put it on to watch *X Factor* as that is a singing show and helium voices somehow don't cut it on a singing competition. I have to say I was shocked at how it sounded. I know that HAs amplify sound but it's never *sounded* like it was amplified before. Now it may as well be coming through a megaphone or bullhorn because that's how it sounds. It's very loud and muffled where the CI sounds so much more natural and clear. Incredible difference!

I have already decided, after just one week, that I will definitely be getting my second ear done sooner rather than later as I had originally planned. My surgeon had suggested three to six months and I think that timing will be about right. I'd like to get this implanted ear a lot better first and then do it. If it's changed this much in a week, I can only imagine what it will be like in six months. At this point, I can't imagine putting my HA in again. It's too bad, too, because it's brand new.

I still have a long way to go but I'm amazed at how far I've come in only one week. I am only on my second program and that was the same as the first program but with more volume.

November 21, 2012 # Week Two

It's been two weeks since my bionic ear was turned on. I heard some new sounds this week. I was walking to a geocache and heard birds. I couldn't see them but I heard them. I went to get the mail and heard a plane overhead. I've heard them before but not for as long as this one. Right after that one flew over, another came overhead. I guess in case I didn't hear the first one. I heard the rain from inside the house. Usually it has to be a torrential downpour for me to hear it, if at all. While I was at a restaurant with my mom, I heard a sound that I didn't recognize. My mom pointed to a lady at another table who was rearranging her leftovers in a bag. Evidently it's *not okay* to smack somebody on the head and tell them to stop that. So I sat patiently while she finished. It was loud.

I went on a couple of field trips this week to hear new sounds. I went to Disney's California Adventure. I still couldn't understand the voices on the rides (that's on my wish list) but I did hear music all over the place. I had no idea there was that much music. We stopped and listened to the street performers and I could even make out the songs they were singing and could tell the differences in the instruments. By the way, I'm not going to add the "Big Bad Wolf" song to my iTunes.

I also went to the Santa Ana Zoo. The animals didn't make very much noise but the freeway next to the zoo did. I also heard the little train coming and the clanging of the bell. What I was most happy to hear was my friend talking to me while I was looking at the animals. And I didn't have to read her lips.

I had my first "mapping" appointment with the audiologist today. That is where they make adjustments to the programs. Now I have to get used to them all over again. I told her I was able to understand an audiobook all the way home from work. That is *huge* for me. She was pretty surprised and said that I might be able to make phone calls now. I told her I already was and I thought she was going to fall off her chair. She had to make a phone call when I was there and I understood everything she said on the phone with her back to me, too.

She said that my positive attitude and willingness to do the rehab was making a huge difference. I told her all of the different rehab work I've been doing and she was very happy that I was putting so much time into it. She hadn't heard about some of the programs so she wrote them down. Hopefully, they will help some other people.

I also talked to the lady that deals with insurance companies. I told her that I'd like to have the other ear done and asked if she knew if my insurance would cover two ears in one year. She said we'd probably have to appeal but that we could do it. I told her I had just gotten a new hearing aid and we both decided that would not sit well with the insurance so I returned it. Now we can show them that it was returned because it doesn't work well, which might help my cause. But now I'm without a hearing aid. I haven't wanted to wear it, but it was nice to have for a security blanket. Oh well. Good riddance to that.

I do rehab every chance I get. It's important to train the brain how to use this new way of hearing. I listen and read along with audiobooks. I have downloaded the Angel Sound program where I listen to different words and have to click on what I think I am hearing. I found a great iPad app called Hear Coach that tests my hearing in different noisy situations. Of course, watching TV helps, too, although I still have to use the captions on that. I have people read words to me that I have to repeat back. That one is really hard to do. I have also joined a supportive email group, and we do phone, music, and listening homework and report back to the group. I am very grateful to that group.

November 26, 2012 # A Wish Came True

I love to hike. I usually hike with my friend, Melissa. Occasionally I go on group hikes with my geocaching friends. Today was a group hike. It was the first hike I've been on since I've gotten the implant. It started out as they usually do. I could understand the person I was hiking right next to as long as I read their lips. I could not understand the other conversations going on around me. This went on for a couple of miles. Then Jeremy joined the group.

We hiked another mile or so and, as we stood around a geocache talking, I noticed that I could easily understand what Jeremy was saying without even looking at him. His voice sounded just like the narrator on the audiobook I've been listening to.

We hiked some more and, on the last mile back, it happened. I was next to Kathy (who sounded like a very young Marcia Brady) and Lee and Jeremy were behind me. All of a sudden, all three of their voices were crystal clear. I could understand every single word that they said without reading any of their lips. It wasn't just one sentence it was the entire conversation. I have never been so happy to hear a conversation about politics before in my life. I got a bit emotional (Okay, okay I was bawling) and poor Kathy stopped because she thought something must be very wrong. I just couldn't believe it was really happening. Lee gave me a big hug and we continued on. The topic switched to tattoos and I could understand that, too. That was probably the best mile I've ever walked.

December 1, 2012 ClearVoice + T-Mic = Another Great Week

At my mapping appointment last week I was given a new program — ClearVoice. This program lessens the sound of constant noise, which is great for places like restaurants. I was also given a thing called a T-Mic which moves the microphone from high on my head to the base of my ear. It makes it so that you can hold a phone in the normal position and also seems to make everything sound richer.

I had a three-hour dinner at Red Robin tonight with a friend and, about halfway through, I realized that I was looking more at her eyes than her mouth. That was a first. I also am pretty sure I didn't use the dreaded "what?" word as often as I used to. It seemed like I could understand much more of what she was saying with a lot less effort on my part. I'm sure it was a whole lot less frustrating for her, too. The funny thing was, she was the one that was complaining about the noise the most.

I've been having a harder time understanding Bob. His voice is a bit deeper than it was and has a weird tone to it that I can't figure out how to describe. I asked him if he would want to work on rehab with me so that I could get used to his new voice. He said no. But when I went upstairs where he was, he had me close my eyes and take about a gazillion deep breaths to get me good and relaxed. Then he started talking to me and I could easily understand what he was saying with my eyes closed. He tried to trick me a few times. He said, "Today is Thursday. Tomorrow is Monday." I caught him, though. Then he sang parts of about six different songs and I got them all. I told him he has to use his "upstairs voice" when he's downstairs from now on because I can understand that.

Mom had a doctor's appointment today and I went with her to that. Her doctor was very soft spoken, but I understood everything he said and didn't have to ask him to speak louder.

I was also able to use the phone in my office. I haven't been able to understand on that phone in years. I always have to get a co-worker to listen to my voicemails for me. To my surprise, the volume was only at the midpoint, not all the way up. My cellphone is much easier to understand using my new ear, too.

My brother, Steve, goes for his final test on Monday to see if he qualifies for an implant. I'm hoping that he will be able to get one very soon.

December 3, 2012 TV and iTunes

It just gets better and better. I turned my iTunes on my computer to listen to music while I worked. I was surprised to find that I needed to turn the volume down to less than the halfway point. I've always had to listen to it at full volume. Music still needs to be greatly improved but I'm happy to recognize the songs. They just don't sound that great yet. Some artists' voices sound better than others.

I turned my soaps on at lunchtime and the closed captioning was all garbled. Normally when that happens I am not able to understand anything. This time, I could understand almost all of what some of the characters said, even the women. Wow! It's so strange, and wonderful, to be able to actually watch the people instead of always reading along. The captions came back on and I started reading along again, but then I stopped doing that and only read when I missed something or when certain characters came on. This is really great.

I also finally heard my cat's bell and tags the other day.

December 11, 2012 Second Mapping / First Test

I went to my second mapping appointment today. That's where they make adjustments to the three programs that I have on my processor. She tested me for the first time since I've had my implant. Wow! Astounding results.

Let me backtrack a little bit so that you can understand the results. With my hearing aids, I had to read lips pretty much 100% of the time. Unfortunately, I'm not perfect and it was pretty much impossible to understand an entire conversation. Sometimes if the setting was perfect (one-on-one with no noise) I would get the majority of it but if there were multiple people around talking to each other it was much harder. I might have understood 50% of a conversation. Now that may sound pretty good to you. But think about hearing a joke. Would you want to listen to just the middle part of a joke and not hear the setup or the punchline? That's what my world was like a lot. If I missed the first part of a conversation then I didn't know what the topic was. Even if I could understand after that, it didn't always help if I didn't know who or what the subject was. I often had to ask somebody what they were talking about. Sometimes it was better to simply go off in my own head and have a conversation with myself.

Let's get back to today's appointment. I went into the soundproof booth for the tests. She did the tone test, which is where you hold a button and she plays a variety of beeps and you press the button each time you hear the beeps. In the past I had tinnitus which is a ringing in the ears. I still have it in my un-implanted side but it's gone on the implanted side if my processor is on. It's very difficult to take that tone test when your ears are ringing because you're not sure if you *really* are hearing something or not. Today it was strange because I had to keep telling myself, "Yes, you're really hearing that". Prior to the implant, I was about as low on the audiogram as it could get. Today, it was actually better than normal at some tones and pretty much normal in others.

Then we came to the sentence testing. That is where they say a variety of sentences with different people speaking them. You have to repeat back what you can understand. Keep in mind there is no lip reading on these tests. It is hearing only. With my hearing aids on I simply sat there. I couldn't make out a single word. In fact, I couldn't hear it and wanted them to turn it up but they said that the speech was at a normal speaking level. Today, I was a little disappointed because I was still missing a lot of each sentence. I was happy that I had the volume to actually be able to hear the sentences, but I still felt like I was straining to understand. Then all of a sudden, it became louder and clearer and I understood the majority of every single sentence. Wow! What a change. It turned out that she did the first half at fifty decibels and I got 69%. Then she upped it to sixty decibels and I got 90%.

Then she did the word test. I was very curious to know how I would do on that one. It was simply fifty random words that you had to repeat back. When I did it with just my hearing aids on before, I got two words right or 4%. Today I got nineteen words right or 38%. But I also got a great deal of portions of the words — i.e. I knew it began with a T, for example, or knew it was an "oo" sound. That wasn't great but it was definitely much improved.

I asked her how many people have the surgery and she said that last year they had about five to seven all year. This year they had five to seven in the past few months. She wants to start a support group with her patients. I told her that I recently signed up to be a Bionic Ear Association (BEA) mentor where I could help people who are thinking about getting an implant or need help along the way. She was happy to hear that I would be willing to help out with that.

She changed my program based on the test results and gave me more volume that I can grow into. I seem to be going through volume pretty quickly. I told her that I was having a hard time in really noisy situations so she added another program for that. I have a geocaching event at a really noisy place tomorrow night so we'll see how that works.

Overall, I'm extremely pleased with how well the implant is working. In the last week or two I've been able to easily understand some people that I had trouble understanding before. I'm beginning to be able to understand the TV without always looking at the closed captions. I can usually understand what people are saying in the front seat of the car if I'm sitting in the back seat. I can hear my iPad now, and I have to turn the volume down quite a bit on other things that had to be full volume before.

I go back for my next mapping appointment in March and we've decided that is when I should probably start the process with the insurance on implanting my other ear.

December 16, 2012 Music and Movies

My brother, Curtis, and his wife, Rebecca, invited me to go see the movie *Argo* with them tonight. This would be my first movie since having the implant. In the past, I loved to go to the movies. Bob and I would go every week as our "hot date." We went for many years. But then my hearing got worse and I couldn't understand the words anymore so we stopped going. My dad loves to go to the movies so I would still go with him from time to time, and others, too, but it had gotten to the point where I could understand maybe fifteen words in a whole movie. Dad loves action movies so if you know who the good guys and the bad guys are you can still enjoy the movie.

We went to Bella Terra which is a nearby outdoor shopping mall. They had a band in the amphitheater and that is where Curtis and Rebecca were when I got there. Listening to bands and music on the radio hasn't been all that great for me either. Sometimes I could figure out what song they were singing and sometimes I could get part of the instruments but it just hasn't been very enjoyable. When I got to where they were, the band wasn't playing. Once they started up, I could hear the instruments very clearly. Then the singer started singing and I could understand every word. I did know the song so it's much easier to understand the words when you know what they are singing — but I *did* hear it very clearly — every word. Good ol' sappy me started bawling again (I really need to stop that!) and poor Rebecca wondered what was wrong. I had already warned Curtis that I might get a little emotional in the movie if I could understand it, but this caught me off guard. I wasn't expecting it to sound that good. He knew what was happening and they were both happy for me.

I realized another thing about music when I was in the car today. I could listen to it as loud as I wanted to. Part of a digital hearing aid's job is to make really loud noises softer and soft noises louder. If you like to crank up the music you really can't because the hearing aids just keep lowering the volume. Today a song came on and I was able to crank up the volume and sing my heart out. I have noticed, too, that my singing has gotten better with the CI. I used to love to sing when I was a kid. I was in the chorus in school, I sang in plays, and I even had solos way back then. But when you can't hear the music very well it's harder to sing in tune.

I got my ticket for the movie and knew they had closed captioning devices there now. It turns out they have had them since August but I didn't know that. I got it and set it up. You put one end firmly into the cup holder and then twist it around so that the little mini screen is where you want it to be. When the movie starts, the words come on the little screen.

Most people automatically think that since I read lips I should be able to get most of the movie by reading the actors' lips. Well, pay attention the next time you go to the movies and you will see just how many words are spoken with no lips shown. You will hear voiceovers, see actors from the sides, from the back, etc. Even when they do show them from the front, it is hard to read their lips. I'm not sure why that is, but it's true.

The movie started with a voiceover narrative. There was no background noise and the woman was very clear. I understood almost every word. Then the action started and it became a bit harder. I noticed movie captioning was not the same as TV captioning. When I watch TV, the captioning lags behind what is being said. That has been horrible for me in the past, but it's actually very good now because it gives me a chance to try to understand what they are saying and, if I can't, I can still read along.

The captioning tonight was very quick and almost ahead of the movie. So I had a choice to either try to understand what the actors were saying or read along. Since I could tell it was going to be a movie with a lot of dialog, I chose to read along. There was one actor, Alan Arkin's Lester, who had a fantastic voice. Whenever he was on, I just listened without reading along and he was great. Dad likes to see the same movies over and over. I may go once with him and read along and, if I like the movie, go again with no captioning and use it for rehab practice.

Seeing the movie tonight and being able to understand every word, even though it was with an assisted listening device, was still a major treat. I'm looking forward to going to more movies and maybe I'll even be able to get Bob to go on "hot dates" again with me to the movies.

December 24, 2012 Christmas Wow

Wow! I stood with my cat, Kenya, on the porch for a second so she could see the lights. I heard jingle bells and looked to see where they were coming from. Next I heard, "Ho, Ho, Ho! Merry Christmas!" I looked down the street and there was Santa Claus going into a neighbor's house. I would have missed him without my bionic ear. I wonder if he's coming here next.

January 1, 2013 # A Week of Wows

My mom is having knee replacement surgery next week. We went to a class at Kaiser to learn about the surgery. Unfortunately, we got there late and the only two seats next to each other were in the very last row at the back of the room. Normally, that would be a very bad thing as I wouldn't be close enough to read lips and definitely not close enough to hear. The presenters did not use a microphone. I was shocked to find that I could understand the physical therapist very clearly and could also understand the majority of what the doctor said, too. People were asking questions from the audience and I couldn't understand them but Mom said she couldn't understand them either. I sure wish I could understand that clearly when I was in college.

I went to see the movie *The Hobbit* at the IMAX 3D. Since I've discovered captioning devices, I asked for one but was told that since it was filmed in the IMAX version no captioning was available. That simply meant that I would be forced to try listening. I was pleasantly surprised that I could understand almost every word the Bilbo Baggins character said and probably half of what the other characters said, too. Prior to having my implant I understood about fifteen words in the entire movie (no exaggeration) and was lucky if I understood a full sentence. It was a real treat to be able to understand as much as I did. I've got a long way to go but I was very pleased.

Tonight was Curtis' New Year's Eve party. I was not expecting to understand much. Noisy parties are usually doomed for me. I was able to turn the volume down low enough that I could have conversations. The best part is that I was actually able to hear the music that was playing. Hearing aids "help" you in that it lowers the volume on loud music. Unfortunately, it lowers it so much that it's never loud enough to be able to dance to it. I would often have to feel vibrations and watch how others were dancing in order to dance myself. Tonight I could hear the music pretty clearly and danced my heart out.

I can tell 2013 is going to be a great year!

January 12, 2013 It's the Little Things

There are lots of little moments with this ear that make me smile. I went into Bob's "man cave" the other night. He was intently watching a movie on his TV, so I looked at it and realized I could understand every single word. He didn't have the captioning on and we didn't turn up the volume. I still have the captioning on when I watch TV and I have been trying to not look at it, but old habits are hard to break and I don't want to miss anything on my shows, so I leave them on. I really probably should start watching some shows that I don't care about with the captioning off. That way if I miss words it won't matter, but at least I'll be practicing more on actively listening than I am now.

Yesterday, Dad read to me from my word lists for rehab. He reads a word and then I say it back. There are "closed sets" of words like "colors" and "months" that were hard for me in the beginning. I sailed through all of those lists. Then there were random words that were harder but I still got most of those fairly easily this time. I had to really concentrate the last time we did those lists a little over a month ago. It was nice to see the change.

My brother, Steve, and I got a pretty good laugh. I gave him the lists and told him that they were easy for me now. His surgery is scheduled for February 8 to get his implant. Anyway, his response was, "Those lists are boring and easy. I had Shirley read them to me and I got every one of them right. Were they *really* actually hard for you?" I told him they were at first. I found it hard to believe that he could understand those words with his hearing aids. I asked him if he was looking at Shirley when she read the lists. He said he was. I pointed out that he wasn't actually "hearing" her at all, but reading her lips, and that if she covered her mouth when she read them, those "easy" words would be a whole lot more challenging. We both laughed at that point when he realized what he had done.

Another "little thing" happened today when I left the office. I was in the almost empty parking lot when I heard my name being called. I looked all over and didn't see anyone so I asked who was calling me and sure enough, a couple of the guys waved from the other end of the parking lot. I never would have heard that before.

It's the "little things" that make my day. I can't wait for Steve to get his fill of "little things" too.

January 24, 2013 A Couple of Things I Don't Miss

My old hearing aids had ear molds. They went deep in the ear and fit snuggly. They didn't hurt, but they sure made my ears itch. Plus, the wax was horrendous. I was always scratching my ears and trying to get the wax out. Every night when I took a shower I had this rubber bulb that I would use to squirt warm water in my ears to keep the wax out. When I had to have the doctor remove the wax from my ears — ouch! That hurt sometimes. With the CI, there are no more molds and . . . no more wax. No more itching either.

I also had tinnitus for as long as I can remember. Tinnitus is when your ears ring. People have the mistaken assumption that if you're deaf or hard of hearing that you must live in a silent world. With tinnitus, it is anything but silent. I had tinnitus the worst I've ever had it for about the last six months before my surgery. It changed from constant light ringing to what sounded liked bells at a railroad crossing or a room full of people clinking their champagne glasses with a fork over and over and over again really, really fast. When it first got that loud I was actually driving with a friend and I asked her who was honking their horn. She said she didn't hear it and asked me to tell her when I heard it again. I did. Nope, she still didn't hear it. It just got worse and worse.

I knew that there was a chance that the tinnitus would go away once I got the CI. In the few weeks after the surgery, but before they turned the implant on, the tinnitus would roar for about thirty seconds to a minute at a time. It was so loud that it actually woke me up from having dreams a couple of times. But I knew that was normal. Lots of people experience that after surgery. Once I was activated, though, it all went away in the ear the CI is on which, thankfully, was my worst tinnitus ear. It is so nice to have actual silence. You just can't imagine how great it is unless you've had that constant 24/7 ringing in your ears. When I take the CI off at night the tinnitus is there sometimes, but not anywhere near as loud as it was, and I only have the CI off when I sleep so it's not a big deal.

I still have the ringing in my left ear, but it's nowhere near as bad as my right ear was, and I'm hoping that will go away when I have my surgery in that ear.

January 31, 2013 It's Waterproof

I had a fantastic massage last night. So good, in fact, that she even gave me a scalp massage. While that feels great, it leaves you looking pretty scuzzy when she's finished. Massage oil gets all over your hair. I definitely had to shower as soon as I got home. That meant I was going to have to dry my hair.

I have long hair. I already use a curling iron so I don't normally like to blow dry it, too. It takes a long time as well. Therefore, I normally shower at night and go to bed with wet hair. Why am I writing about this? For most people wet hair is not a big deal. For people that wear hearing aids, if your hair is wet, you are deaf. It's just that plain and simple. The longer it takes to dry your hair, the longer you can't hear. Thus, showering right before I go to bed solves that problem.

This also means that I tend to avoid situations where my hair is going to be wet for any length of time. I don't like to go in swimming pools or on water rides at amusement parks, for example. Not because I don't like them, but because that means I'm going to have wet hair for a long time, which means no hearing during that time. That also means no conversations.

I was pretty hungry when I got home from my massage. I was expecting a phone call, and a show I wanted to watch was about to come on. I realized, when I was washing my hair, that my Neptune processor was waterproof. For the first time since I was a teenager, I could actually hear with wet hair. I got out of the shower, popped it on my head, ate my dinner, and watched my show — all without having to dry my hair first.

Now I'm looking forward to going swimming in a pool with my friends. When the weather gets warmer I'll wear my waterproof headpiece to California Adventure and go on the rapid ride. By the way, this is one of the reasons why (although not the only reason) I chose the Advanced Bionics brand of implants. They are the only company with a fully waterproof implant.

February 14, 2013 Yuma, Arizona Wows

I went to Yuma, Arizona with my cousin, Sue, for a few days. We love to go geocaching and there was a big event there with 1,200 geocachers. If you don't know what geocaching is, it's basically like an Easter egg hunt. You use a GPS to find geocaches (caches) that are hidden. You find them, sign your name on the piece of paper that's inside the container, and put it back for the next person to find. Go to geocaching.com if you want to see all of the geocaches near you. We cached for several days and had lots of fun.

I picked Sue up at the Irvine train station and then I drove us to Yuma. It's about a four hour drive. It was *awesome* to be able to understand the majority of what she said. In my hearing aid days, she would have had to wear a microphone that would have transmitted her voice into my hearing aids. Otherwise, I would have had to try to keep looking at her to read her lips while she talked. That's not easy to do that and drive for four hours. That alone was a huge relief. People used to get pretty hoarse having to talk loudly to me for that long, too. I'm sure she was able to speak in her regular voice.

When we got to the first cache she read the description to me as she always does. Normally, I would get some of it but would usually have to read it again myself, or stop and read it to myself as she was reading aloud.

Surprisingly, I was able to understand everything she said as I was driving up to it. That was so nice. We went to sixty-eight caches on this trip. For her to be able to read the descriptions while I drove, and be able to understand what she said was really a great thing.

The first night we were there we met up with a couple of our friends and we did some night caching. Normally, that would mean that I would not understand the conversations in the car. Not only were they talking from the back seat, but it was also dark, which meant there was no way I could try to read their lips either. To my surprise, I understood all three of them very clearly. That was something that was on my "wish list" and it was great to be able to check that off.

The big event was on Sunday. They had a guy on the loudspeaker making announcements throughout the day. Before, I would never be able to understand anything he said. This time, depending on where I was sitting, I understood him quite well. They had a big raffle and I had eleven tickets. In the past, someone would have had to listen to them call the numbers and help me with it. Not this time. I could understand the numbers pretty clearly. I didn't win the raffle, but I definitely felt like a winner!

I sure wish I didn't get so darn emotional every time these "wow" moments sneak up on me. Fortunately, I had warned Sue about it ahead of time so she knew nothing was wrong with me when I cried. I'm just so grateful that these miracles just keep coming.

February 20, 2013 # Another Wish Fulfilled

I am a Stampin' Up! demonstrator. I teach people how to make greeting cards and other items using decorative rubber stamps. I've been doing this for twenty years. Once a month I have a Stamp Night in my home for my customers. I also get together with other demonstrators once a month to stamp.

Unfortunately, you have to actually look down at the stamps and what you are stamping on in order to stamp. It's pretty difficult to read lips and stamp at the same time. I have missed out on all of the conversations that go on around me if I'm stamping. It can be a pretty lonely experience when everyone else is laughing and having a good time. I do love stamping, though. I love my customers and stamping friends, too.

Way up high on my hearing wish list is to be able to understand conversations while I am stamping. Tonight was Stamp Night. It was a very small group tonight. Only three customers came. For the most part, those three ladies are pretty quiet. Even so, I didn't actually expect to understand them while I stamped. I've had other Stamp Nights since being activated but haven't really been able to understand the conversations yet. Towards the end of the night tonight, it happened. I was busy working away on my card when all of a sudden I could understand everything that all three of them were saying to each other. I was ecstatic!

This was not a typical Stamp Night with a lot of people all talking and stamping at the same time but I'll take it. It's a start and it has given me hope.

I was also able to understand Bob clearly in the dark this morning. No reading lips there, either.

March 7, 2013 A Big Day for the Husting Family – Steve's Activation and a Memorial Service

It was a very big day for my family. My brother, Steve, started his new life with a cochlear implant today. I was fortunate enough to get to witness the miracle with his wife, Shirley. The three of us went to Kaiser in Los Angeles for his activation. It went as well as I could possibly have hoped for. Steve could hear! Speech is strange for him, as expected, and he said that I sound like R2D2 from *Star Wars*. He said that he could understand words when he read lips. I wanted to test him without reading my lips but he wasn't ready to try that yet. I wasn't sure exactly what he could do. He heard lots of sounds that he hasn't heard in a while: his knuckles rapping on the desk, the shuffling of papers, the elevator ding, my shoes as I was walking in the hallway, sounds of a very faint fountain, the car blinker, and even the radio. Most of all, he could hear our voices and we no longer have to speak loudly to him. This is a habit that's going to be hard to break.

After the activation we went to a really cool book store in Los Angeles called The Last Bookstore. If you are ever in Los Angeles, I highly recommend it. It had a lot of really cool things to look at there. We spent about an hour walking around looking at all of the interesting things. Every now and then Steve would smile as he heard us walking or making other noises.

After that we went to a funeral for a very dear woman, Marilyn Rodeheffer. She is my sister-in-law, Lynn's, mother. It was a sad time for us, as it always is saying a final goodbye to a special loved one. Since this is a book about my hearing journey, I will tell you how it went from my listening perspective. The room was filled with loud music as we came in. At least it was loud to me, but evidently, not to my hearing family, nor to Steve. I enjoyed listening to it, though. The ceremony was very nice. It was especially astonishing for me to be able to understand the majority of what was said without having to concentrate, and without having to read lips. I can't tell you how great it is to be able to look at a speaker in the eyes instead of always concentrating on their mouths. Marilyn was my brother, Brian's, mother-in-law and he gave a very moving speech. I was able to understand every word, and it was a very fitting tribute to a woman who loved him very much. When it came time for the prayer, another "wow" moment came for me. It was the first time that I have been able to bow my head, and even close my eyes, as I listened and understood the prayer all the way through. I have always had to read the lips of the speaker in the past. For me, it was a very moving ceremony. I was grateful to be able to hear it and pay my respects to a woman that meant a lot to me.

The family and a few close friends of Lynn's went to dinner afterwards. Since it was fairly early, we had the place to ourselves. Although it was a large group, there was little background noise other than the people talking at our table. We were all happy (and amazed) to see Steve talking so much to one of Lynn's friends who was sitting across from him. It was a good dinner.

Afterwards, Steve, Shirley and I drove home. Steve was driving and I was sitting behind him. I guess Steve must have built up his confidence after a day of hearing with his new ear because he was finally ready to do some rehab.

He asked me to say the days of the week in random order, of course. He got all but one. We moved on to months and he got all but one then, too. I decided to try something harder. As we drove, Shirley and I would pick out a word from various signs and say them to him. He was to look for what he thought he heard and repeat them back. He did incredibly well at this. He understood probably 90% and we gave him a *lot* of words. He was able to do exactly what I was able to do on my activation day — no more and no less. I was ecstatic! He thought he would be able to do it with his hearing aid, too, and I told him that wasn't possible. He turned his hearing aid on and, sure enough, he wasn't able to get days, months, or words from signs. Earlier in the day, he said that he didn't know what the big deal was because it was just like getting a new hearing aid. I think he now understands that a CI is anything but that. A whole new world is just beginning for him and I am grateful that I was able to share in the first "wow" moments. I am looking forward to many more for him.

March 15, 2013 Second Ear Approved

I just got word that the insurance approved the surgery for my second ear. Yay! I have two expectations for hearing with two ears (bilateral): directionality and better hearing in noise. Believe me, I'm not complaining about the awesome ear I have now, but there are some improvements that can be made. Right now, people call my name, and I can hear them, but I can't tell where they are calling me from. It's also still hard to hear in some noisy places. I normally try to sit so that the people I want to talk to the most are not sitting on my deaf side but that's not always the case. I'm pretty excited.

I'm hoping they will be able to do it the week of April 15th. Keep your fingers crossed for me.

March 28, 2013 # This and That

My surgery has been scheduled for April 22nd at 10:00 am. I have no anxiety or worries about it. I've had enough surgeries to know that the surgeons and staff know what they are doing and will take good care of me. The time is going to fly because I've got a full plate between now and then.

I had another mapping on the 20th. That is when they make adjustments to my processor. I have three different programs that they can do different things with. They made some pretty big adjustments this time. The internal implant has two different ways that the electrodes can work: sequential (S) or paired (P). I'm not sure exactly how they work but it has to do with how the electrodes relate to the ones around them. Anyway, it's kind of like having two separate internal implants. They sound that different. I have been using S all along and I wanted to try out P. So she put that in one of my slots. She also changed my input dynamic range (IDR). IDR is the amount of sound that I have access to. It is not the same as volume. Imagine a window. If the window is only slightly open, you may only see the grass in the backyard. Open the window more and you may discover there is also a tree. Open it even wider and you can see the mountains in the distance. Now imagine the same thing with sound. Well, she opened my window wider. I moved from 60 db to 70 db on both my S and P programs. I told her I was still having a hard time in restaurants so she kept me at the lower IDR and removed lower tones. She said that background noise normally comes from those tones. She also gave me ClearVoice High on that program, which filters out even more constant sounds.

The next day I started a mini vacation. I drove for three hours to my Aunt Edith's home in Buellton. This gave me a chance to try out my car stereo with the new maps. Normally, a new map is like taking a step backwards to get two steps forward. It can take some time to get used to, and it is not unusual to wish you had your old program at first. Well, that was true with the stereo. I could not hear my music as well as I could before the new map. I decided to try the P program and see if that was better. At first it sounded like a lot of static or "out of focus" as someone else described it. I guess it's quite a switch for the brain to get used to. After a couple of songs, it settled in and I actually liked it better. I kept it on that program until I reached Aunt Edith's.

I switched it back to S and she sounded very, very high like quite the munchkin. I switched it back to P to see if she sounded any different. She did. She had a richer sound and was a little more normal but definitely not her old voice. I kept that on for a couple of hours and then switched back to S. Oh boy was that bad. But the brain quickly adapted and she wasn't as bad but still high pitched. S speech is much clearer but the sound seems to be better with P. I know that I need to give both a real chance and am going to have to put P on for a full week without switching back and forth to really see what I think. For now I'm giving the new S map a chance.

I went to San Luis Obispo after seeing Aunt Edith for a few hours. I stayed with an old friend, Sue, for a couple of nights. We hiked on three different trails and saw really beautiful scenery. As you can imagine when two old friends get together there was nonstop talking. At one point I realized how easy it was to understand her (even on the trails) and that I only asked her to repeat herself a couple of times during my whole stay.

After leaving that Sue, I drove down to Santa Barbara and stayed with my cousin, Sue, for another couple of days. We went geocaching one day and then we picked up Aunt Edith. Sue drove us on an incredible mountain road to see the wildflowers. They were spectacular. Even more spectacular was the fact that I could clearly understand Aunt Edith in the backseat behind me the entire time. We have gone on caching trips before where my mom and Aunt Edith were in the backseat talking nonstop and I could never understand anything they said. Oh how I wished Mom could have been with us on this trip. I caught myself smiling many times, not because of the sensational view, but because I could understand her so well.

After leaving Sue's, I drove about an hour to the Ronald Reagan Library. They had a Disney exhibit that I was really wanting to see, and it was just a short detour off the freeway. I was pleased to see that the car stereo sounded good again on the S program. By now, my brain had almost a week to get used to it. I had a "wow" moment at the Library. I didn't have a lot of time to spend there and, as I was quickly going through the Ronald Reagan exhibits, I realized that I was understanding everything that was being said on a nearby video screen. I wasn't looking at it or even actively paying attention to it. It was just background noise, but I was fully comprehending what was being said. That caught me quite off guard in a very good way. I went into the next room and, sure enough, I could understand those videos, too. Pretty cool! There wasn't anybody else in those rooms with me so there was no other background noise at the time. I had lunch with another cousin, Merilee, after I left there. I really need to learn how to control my emotions better because I was telling Merilee about this unexpected pleasure and got a bit choked up. I tend to do that when I can do something that I couldn't do before, or at least for a *very* long time.

It was a fantastic trip. I'm heading to Mexico next week for my brother, Curtis', wedding. I am hoping the weather is warm enough that we can go swimming. I can't wait to try out my waterproof processor and actually hear in the water.

April 13, 2013 Advanced Bionics Visit / Mentoring

I signed up to be a volunteer mentor with Advanced Bionics' Bionic Ear Association (BEA). Many people who are thinking about getting a cochlear implant like to be able to talk to people that have one. It was a huge turning point for Steve and me when we got to meet Al and his wife, Debbie. Al has a CI. I went from worried to very excited in one hour after meeting with them. I knew I wanted to help people just like they helped us.

On the mentoring questionnaire they had a box for "public speaking." I've always loved giving speeches so I told them I would be happy to give speeches. I was quickly asked if I would like to go to Advanced Bionics (AB) in Valencia, CA and give a speech to their employees. They have a "Connect to Patient" program. I was honored to be asked and was grateful to have a chance to let the employees know how much the CI meant to me. Of course, I said yes. I think this is a really great program. It is tedious work making the implants and, of course, I imagine we all feel like our job is just a job every now and then. I think it is really great for them to get to see the miracle that they are a part of, and remind them how important their "job" really is. Not just the manufacturing employees, either, but all of them. They are all important.

I went to Valencia on Wednesday afternoon and stayed the night. Since getting my CI, I have met a lot of other CI users on the Hearing Journey forum online and on Facebook but I hadn't met any of my new friends in person yet. Well, it turns out one of them, Deb McClendon Deitz, happened to have flown in from Texas just a few hours after I got there. She was staying at the hotel right next to mine. We wound up having a five-hour meal and I felt like I've known her all my life.

Since CIs are medical devices, everything they do has to be approved by the FDA. In order to get FDA approval they have to undergo clinical trials. Deb is one of the lucky ones that has been a guinea pig in those clinical trials. She gets to try out the great new, top secret, programs that the company is working on. She visits AB and they run lots of tests on her. The bad part for her is that she doesn't get to keep what she tries out. But at least she knows what is coming. She had a sparkle in her eyes and a giant smile when she told me how great the new software is. Of course, that was all she was able to tell me, no matter how much wine I tried to ply her with. I may ask to see if they can use me in clinical trials some day. I think that would really be interesting to do.

One of the reasons I chose Advanced Bionics is because they *do* continually upgrade the CI. When something new comes out, we just go to the audiologist and they plug the processor into a computer and load up the new software. Some improvements are hardware related. I'll be getting a new device later this year. But many are simply software upgrades. It's a great relief to know that I will be able to keep up with new technology for many years to come.

On Thursday, I gave my speech two times — once in the morning for the regular employees and once in the afternoon for the manufacturing employees. My speech was forty-five minutes and then they had a Q&A period afterwards. My sister-in-law, Shirley, and I made thank you cards for the employees that came to the speech. They seemed to like getting those. I did get choked up a couple of times and I guess, I got the audience crying, too, at one point. The highlight for me was the lady that came up to me afterwards and asked me about my insurance. She told me that her husband was deaf and that she thought he could benefit from a CI. She was under the mistaken impression, as I originally was, that it would be too expensive. In my speech I mentioned that insurance pays for implants so I was very happy that my speech had an impact on her. I think I also made a geocacher out of one of the engineers.

After my morning speech, I was given a tour of the manufacturing floor. There are five floors in the massive building. They employ around five hundred people at that location and many more all over the world. The tour was fascinating. I saw the patent wall where they have plaques of all of the patents that they have. It was very impressive. The T-Mic and the Aqua Mic are patented by AB so their competitors can't make those features. The T-Mic is a microphone at the opening of the ear instead of on top of the ear. It allows me to hold a phone up to my ear like a normal person and I can wear headphones and earbuds. The Aqua Mic is the fully waterproof piece. Only AB has a fully waterproof processor.

I was amazed at how clean everything is required to be. The employees had to wear hair nets, booties, sanitize their hands, and then put gloves on *and* wear a jumpsuit over their clothes and no makeup. Everything is made by hand and they have to do all of their work using microscopes since the electrodes are as thin as strands of hair. I can't tell you the details of what I saw and heard or they would have to kill me, but I will say that I was *very* impressed and amazed by the whole thing.

A small group of students that are learning to be sign language interpreters came to my afternoon speech. I was able to sit with them for about a half hour before my speech and answered their questions and showed them what my CI looked like. I really enjoyed talking to them and I may see if any local colleges would like me to speak to their students in the same program.

I have been enjoying being a mentor. I have emailed numerous people and I finally got to meet one in person today. It was really great to be able to talk to her and put her mind at ease about things. Hopefully, I was able to get her past the worried stage and into the excited stage.

By the way, my surgery was changed to April 23rd — just ten days to go!

April 16, 2013 Goodbye to Old Hearing – Trying my Hearing Aid One Last Time

I have one week to go until surgery, which means this is the final week I will ever be able to wear a hearing aid and listen the "old" way. I was activated five months ago and have only worn my hearing aid a couple of times since then and just for a couple of minutes. I knew I didn't like it before when I tried it but I still wanted to try it one more time.

I put it on while I was watching TV. Then I remembered that I couldn't hear the TV before. I had to use my Bluetooth device that streamed the sound from the TV directly into my hearing aids. I got that out and turned it on. The sound was still so faint that I had to read the captioning or I missed what was said. It's funny because I knew I had to do that before but I guess it didn't really dawn on me just how deaf I was (well, still am when my CI is off). I also thought sound would be more "normal" through my hearing aid. It turns out that it is just different.

Then I tried my iPad, which I couldn't hear at all. I forgot about that. I then tried a song I've been listening to on YouTube. Nope, it was not loud enough. I'd forgotten about that, too. I tried my iTunes on my computer at full blast and barely got that. I also tried my phone — nope. When I was with my audiologist yesterday, she was making some changes to my CI and I had to read her lips. That was taking a bit of effort to do. I haven't been having to do very much lip reading lately, so I'm out of practice.

It really is pretty awesome that I am able to hear the TV, my iPad, iTunes, YouTube and my phone through my CI. The volume is at about the halfway mark which is just like normal people. I can also understand many shows without reading the captioning and didn't need it at all at the last movie I went to. I knew this was a miracle, but I guess I have been taking it for granted because I completely forgot what it really sounded like before I had the CI.

I am ready to go full steam ahead with my new ear. That ear was actually my "good" ear, if there was such a thing, so I'm curious to know how it does in comparison to my first ear. The first time I was told to wear the CI without the hearing aid to force my brain to use it and get used to it. I didn't miss my hearing aid very much and now I know why. There really wasn't anything to miss. I know that if I really want to give my second ear the best possible chance that I need to wear it by itself to force my brain to use it. I think that is going to be much more difficult because I will definitely miss the CI ear.

I would like to hear my mom's voice one more time with the hearing aid but I have a feeling it won't be the same. Bob sounds a lot different than I remember him sounding. I'm glad I put the hearing aid back on because I will no longer long for the old sounds because, quite frankly, they don't sound very good. Not only is everything too low in volume but the sound quality is poor, too. I am reminded of the first day I was activated with the CI. I was having lunch in a restaurant with my parents and I remember telling my mom that she was now "in my ear" and not "out there." I was getting much better sound even on that very first day.

Voices are still not right but I'm told it can take a year or longer for that to happen. I've been reminded that I am still a baby "CI-borg" and that I need to have patience. I'm okay with that. I would keep the clarity that I've been given, over regular voices any day of the week.

I'm excited to get my second ear turned on. It's only been six months since my last surgery but I don't remember what it's like to hear in two ears anymore. I haven't missed my other ear. When I wore two hearing aids, I would be devastated if one of my hearing aids went out, but that hasn't been the case with the CI. I know it is supposed to be much better with two because people who have two keep telling me that. The second ear will be turned on in about a month. It's going to be a wild ride!

April 24, 2013 Second CI Surgery

I had my second CI surgery yesterday. I had what is called a "rock star" surgery — no pain, no nausea, no dizziness, no loss of taste — nothing. They put this big ol' cone on the side of my head and they strap it on. They folded my non-surgery ear in half and put the strap over that. That hurt. I finally figured out what they did and was able to unfold it. Yeesh!

I can't drive yet, and I'm sleeping a lot, but the only pain pill I have taken is a Tylenol. I do hear loud roaring tinnitus from time to time but it doesn't last long and I know that is normal. It will go away when I'm activated.

Now comes the hard part — having enough patience to wait three weeks until they turn my ear on!

May 5, 2013 Recovery After Surgery

I'm pretty much back to normal. That is if anyone can ever really say I was ever normal. I had hives and bumps. I wasn't too alarmed about the hives because I had that after the first surgery, too. That time we passed it off as an allergy to a new soap I was using. But I haven't used that since the last surgery so we decided I must be allergic to the Neosporin that Bob was putting on the incision. The surgeon stopped having us use the Neosporin and the hives stopped, too. It took a little longer for the bumps to go away but they are gone now.

I do have loss of taste again. It's a little more severe this time but maybe that's because it's been added to the loss from before. Who knows? It's not bad. It is most noticeable with sweet foods, which is probably a good thing because maybe I won't want to eat as many. Water tastes different, too, but not bad. Sometimes breads are a bit bland and dry.

I didn't have any pain, never had to take any pain meds, and the above symptoms were the worst — so I'll take it. I see my surgeon on Thursday.

I get activated on May 15th. It seems like it is going very slowly. My brother, Steve, says patience is not my strong suit and I guess he's right about that. I do think it will be interesting to see what it will sound like this time. I think it will make me appreciate how far I've come with the first one because I do think I will notice a big difference. It's going to take time for the volume to get back up and for voices to catch up to this one. If I can stand it, I will try to only wear the new one for a while by itself, but I have a feeling that might be too hard to do. I am also persistent and determined. Hopefully, my persistence and determination will override my impatience in that area.

May 14, 2013 Advanced Bionics Testing

They turn on my new ear tomorrow morning! Yay! It seems like forever between surgery and activation, so I was happy when Advanced Bionics contacted me and asked me if I would like to help out their R&D team for a couple of days. Of course I said yes.

On Sunday afternoon I drove up to Valencia and cached (is there anything else?). It was 97 degrees. I must be crazy. Then on Monday and today I met with the people there and did some top secret, I'll have to kill you if I tell you, stuff. I can't tell you what I did or saw, but I can say that it was pretty exciting for me.

Where I work, we design and manufacture R/C cars. To a lot of people that doesn't mean a whole lot. But ask a guy that is into R/C cars if he wants to come in and talk to the engineers and work on top secret stuff that hasn't been released yet and you can bet he'd be excited.

What I guess I'm trying to say is, it was pretty cool to be asked. I *can* tell you that I was very impressed by the people I met and how many people they have just working on new hardware/software for us. These things can take years to come to fruition so their dedication is pretty phenomenal. It gave me a lot of hope for my future, too. You can't beat that.

I had Monday afternoon free, and had planned on caching again, but it was 101 degrees and I draw the line at 100 degrees. I have my limits you know. I went and saw the movie, *42,* instead — great choice. It was a good movie. I got the special captioned glasses but I didn't need them. I understood probably 97% of the movie all on my own. I know I've said it before, but it thrills me to death when that happens and it seems to be happening more and more often, too.

I'm back at home now and in about thirteen hours I will have a second ear.

May 15, 2013 Activation #2

My activation appointment was at 8:30 this morning to turn my second ear on. I woke up at 4:45 am and couldn't get back to sleep. At probably about 5:15 am I started crying uncontrollably. I think it finally sunk in that I was actually going to have two ears again. It finally seemed real.

I picked up my friend, Marsha, and we headed to see my audiologist, Cheryl. There were two students in there with her today. When she introduced me, she told them that I had only been activated on my other ear for six months. All of a sudden I turned into a celebrity and they said, "Oh! You're the one everybody's talking about!" She didn't say *what* they were talking about but I guessed it wasn't about my fashion sense. I got a kick out of that.

Then they fired up the electrodes. There are sixteen electrodes implanted in my head. She turned them all on at once and got to a certain comfort level in volume and then they worked on segments of four electrodes at a time. When she first turned it on, I didn't realize I was hearing people talk. I thought we were on the "beep" part of the setup. When they are working on the volume, you hear a few beeps and then they make it louder or softer and you hear more beeps, etc. The beeps are different pitches. Then I realized that the beeping that I was hearing was actually us talking. I know that it is common for people to only hear the beeps when they are first activated and I had prepared myself for that. When my brother, Steve, was activated he said that I sounded like R2D2. But as she went on trying to get to a comfortable volume, I all of a sudden understood what she was saying and speech became speech.

We went on with the testing and they sounded like Alvin and the Chipmunks or Munchkins from *The Wizard of Oz* but I sounded very deep like a man. I didn't like that at all. I asked her what strategy they had me on — S or P. The electrodes can interpret speech two different ways. I have been using S on my other ear and have had great success in speech recognition. I did try the P strategy and liked it better for voices but speech was not as clear. It turns out they had me on P so they switched it to S. I liked that a lot better.

When we were all done, there was some kind of computer glitch and they thought they had lost all of the programming that they had just done. At this point I was turned off, which means I was completely deaf and could only read their lips. Marsha told me there was a problem and I could understand what they were saying, but figured we would just start over if that was the case, so I wasn't really concerned about it. I was just happy I could understand speech again.

I had agreed to give a testimonial on my surgeon. I met with a lady in his office for an interview after the activation. I was very pleased that I was able to understand her so well. I was lip reading, but I did understand what she was saying with only the new ear on.

Then I took Marsha back home. On the way, I had her pick out words from signs to tell me and then I repeated back to her what I thought she said. I was able to pick out the words most of the time until she would do trick questions and read from a car or signs on the other side of the road. I think my brothers must have trained her. In any case, I was pleased about that.

When I got back home I had to go to work (I work from home a few days a week). I turned on Pandora on my iPhone. I plugged one end of the cord in to the phone and the other end into my processor. The sound then goes directly into my ear much like wearing earbuds. That music was only going into the new ear and not the old one. I was very surprised that I could understand a lot of the commercials. It took months to get to that point on my other ear and here I was able to do it on the first day. Wow! I was also picking up some lyrics on songs I didn't know, which is also unheard of on the first day.

Another big plus is that my tinnitus is finally gone! No more ringing in my ears when my processors are on my head. If I take them off, the ringing is there, but I only take them off when I go to bed. That alone is worth having the surgery. It is such a huge relief.

My routine for a while will be to do rehab on the new ear. I went to the library and got some audiobooks. I will listen and read along to them. I will also watch videos, do phone exercises and the Angel Sound program which is mostly picking words that I think I am hearing. There are also many iPad apps that I will use, as well as going to movies, etc. In order to get the most out of this ear, I have to use it by itself, at the very least during rehab, but it is better if I can do it even more. It definitely has to have a chance to catch up to the first one. I was pretty amazed at how far the first one has come.

May 16, 2013 Music in Stereo

I can see I'm going to need to invest in Kleenex stock. I bawled my fool head off all the way to work today. I was driving the Porsche and popped in a Styx CD (one of my favorite bands of all time). I was *not* expecting the result I got.

Let me give you a little background first. Before my first surgery, when I was only wearing hearing aids, I pretty much stopped listening to music in the Porsche. I could barely make out what song was playing and it sounded horrible. After I got my first ear it got much better. I could easily tell what song was on and I could understand the lyrics if it was a song I knew. I was beginning to even understand lyrics on songs I didn't know. However, I was having a problem with road noise. It was too loud. In order to get rid of road noise, I had to turn on a program on my processor that helps to lower that (ClearVoice) and then I lowered my IDR, too. IDR is how much sound the CI is letting in. Well what that did was, it either made vocals clearer or instruments more prominent, but not both. So I was sacrificing something to try to get rid of the road noise and make music better.

Today, however, with both ears turned on, the road noise was practically nonexistent. Then I decided to try the highest IDR I have which is 80 IDR (I usually use 60 in the car). There was still no problem with road noise. I'm listening to Styx and it didn't take long to remember what stereo sounds like. Wow! I can't believe I forgot how incredible that is. I got *all* of the instruments plus the vocals and no road noise *and* stereo sound. Different speakers play different things and music was all around me. I was in heaven. I have to admit, I didn't want to leave the car when I got to the office. Also, I'm actually looking forward to the 45-60 minute drive home. I never thought I'd say that.

So that is one *huge* wish list item checked off.

May 23, 2013 Week One of Ear Two

It's been a very busy week with lots of different listening opportunities. I went to the office on Thursday, Friday, and Tuesday. I wore both ears. That said, however, I am a firm believer in rehabbing the new ear, which means it needs to be stimulated as much by itself as possible. In the mornings, I hooked up my processor and my iPhone to "direct connect" mode. That is, I connected them with a cable that allowed sound from my phone to go directly into my ear, much like wearing an ear bud would sound like. I didn't have any music or audiobooks loaded, so I listened to the Pandora app on Thursday. Pandora is like a personal radio. You can have "stations" that are made up of music that you like. You can choose from various genres or you can create your own custom stations. I like Kelly Clarkson and Carrie Underwood so I made a station suggesting those two singers. It then plays music of similar styles. I also have a Maroon 5 station. In my old ear, those stations sound fantastic. In my new ear, well, not so much. Since they are not songs that I know, the vocals sounded like screeching cats and it sounded like the singers were screaming every lyric. The instruments sounded good, though. I put up with that for about an hour until I couldn't stand it anymore, then I looked for free audiobooks. I downloaded *A Christmas Carol* and listened to that. That turned out to be pretty fun because it was all in British accents. By lunchtime, I was speaking with a British accent myself. My brother, Curtis, however, was a Scrooge and told me if I kept it up he was going to throw me out of the car.

On Friday and Tuesday, I had Elton John loaded up. Since I know the words and melodies to all of those songs, they actually sounded quite good — no more screeching cats. On a couple of the songs, his voice even sounded the way I remembered. Needless to say, I teared up when I heard that. It's pretty remarkable when that happens. It gives me hope.

In the afternoons at the office, I wore just the new ear for about an hour. I listened to the sounds around me. People sounded like the RX-24 robot on the Star Tours ride at Disneyland. I could understand what they were saying, but they were high pitched robot sounds. Strangely enough, one of my co-workers stood outside my door and talked to me to see if I could understand her. I asked her to slow down and I did understand what she was saying. When I told her I was just wearing the new ear, her jaw dropped to the floor. I definitely couldn't do that on the second day with the first ear.

When I am at home, I listen with only the new ear. I do an hour of solid rehab every night. I do a half hour of reading along while listening to the

Dean Koontz *The Taking* audiobook and then I do a phone exercise, an audio exercise, and various word exercises. I also watch TV with just the new ear. I am surprised that I am able to understand some people without captions, but mostly I need the captions. I am also shocked at the scores I am getting on some of the rehab programs. I am actually able to understand some of the words that I am hearing. It took me a couple of months to get to that point with the first ear.

Thursday nights are family dinner nights. It was a big group this time. Normally, I try to sit to the left since I only had my right ear to listen out of. Now it doesn't matter. Yay! This time I sat in the middle. Before, if I sat in the middle, and the people were talking on my right that I didn't want to hear because I wanted to listen to the people in front of me or to my left, it was difficult to understand them. This time, however, I was able to easily focus on anyone anywhere at the table. The other people could have their conversations and they did not dominate my ears. It was great.

I am a Stampin' Up! demonstrator. I sell rubber stamps and I teach people how to make greeting cards and other items using stamps. On Saturday, I went to my upline, Sandy's, meeting. There were over sixty demonstrators there. During the first part of the meeting, we mill around looking at cool displays and we watch demonstrations of the products. The meeting is held at The Spaghetti Factory which has wooden floors. Add in all of the talking of sixty demonstrators and, well, it is *loud*. Fortunately, Advanced Bionics has a program for our processors called Clear Voice that filters out some noise. Unfortunately, I do not have that on my new ear yet. Hearing out of my old ear sounded fine, but the new ear got every sound including the droning of the air conditioner. When people tried to talk to me I definitely had to resort to reading lips and uttering the dreaded "what?" word.

Then the meeting portion began. Normally, I have to sit right in front of the person speaking so that I can read their lips. This time, however, I sat with my friends at our table a little distance away from the people speaking. I was able to get the majority of what they said. They did use a microphone and that sound was not good but, at one point, they forgot about the microphone and I actually understood them very easily. It turns out that my sister-in-law said that she, too, had a hard time understanding what they were saying when they were using the microphone, and that it was much easier when they didn't.

Cool! I did listen to Sandy with both ears (she sounded good), then with the old ear (she sounded like a man), and with the new ear (she sounded like Donald Duck). I was able to understand the conversations at our table during lunch after the meeting, even the conversations at the opposite end of the table.

Sunday was one of my favorite events of the year. It was MouseAdventure at Disneyland. MouseAdventure is an all day "race" made up of various "quests" (puzzles) that you have to go all over Disneyland to solve. There are four members of our team, two of which I have played with for years. Teams have to stay together at all times. You can't send somebody off to go check something out. It is not unusual for me to lead the team to the next location only to have someone tug at me and then I turn around and realize the team has stopped. I was hoping that this time they could simply call my name, but it was too noisy for me to hear them. One really cool thing did happen though. At one point there was a mob of teams scouring a bulletin board looking for a clue. We knew that the clue was in that area so we went over there, too. As soon as we got there, Doris reached over and whispered in my ear, "Look at the chest at the base of the tree." Sure enough, there was the clue that everyone was looking for. Right there in front of their eyes, yet no one saw it but Doris. Even more incredible to me, was that I understood her. You see, any time anyone has whispered to me in the past, I have always had to stop them and tell them that they needed to face me. They could still whisper, but I had to read their lips in order to understand what they were saying. So for me to be able to understand her was *huge*.

On Monday, I went to "Lunch Club." Once a month I get together with about a dozen of my fellow Stampin' Up! demonstrators and we stamp all day. Typically, that involves a bunch of chatter that I don't understand. I look down when I stamp and I can't read lips. At the last Lunch Club that I went to in March, I was able to understand some of what was being said around me. This time, I understood what was being said *and* I figured out who was saying it. With two ears, I am able to finally figure out where sound is coming from. I even tried to differentiate between their voices and I was able to do that a little bit, too. I even got part of a conversation that was going on in the room next to us. All eleven of us sat around the table at lunchtime and I was able to understand all of the conversations around the table, too.

Yesterday, I spent the day caching with my friend, Deb. Although this isn't new now, it is always so nice to be able to understand my passenger while I am driving. Deb had a *very* exciting story to tell me and I was really happy that I was able to understand what she said. We stopped for lunch at that point so that she could tell me the rest without being interrupted by caches. Deb is an aspiring writer who has now gotten interest from an agent. She told me the story of the fictional book she is writing and it definitely sounds like a winner. I wouldn't be surprised if they turn her book into an Academy Award-nominated movie. You heard it here first. Deb Boone is going to be known worldwide some day. An interesting observation that Deb made was that I was pronouncing my consonants much crisper and clearer. I do listen to an awful lot of words in my rehab, and have to distinguish the difference in those sounds without reading lips, so maybe that is changing the way I speak, too.

I have noticed that voices are changing with this ear. The audiobook lady isn't as annoying as she was in the beginning, and she is getting a bit deeper. I am very much looking forward to my next mapping in a week. I will have Clear Voice medium added to my processor. That program should cut out a lot of annoying sounds like computer fans, road noise, air conditioner hums, refrigerator hums, etc.

For now a new week has begun. I wonder what "wow"s this week holds in store?

May 27, 2013 First Swim Today

My brother, Steve, and I went for a swim in the community pool at his housing complex today. I haven't been able to hear while swimming in a pool for about thirty years. I am not sure if Steve has *ever* been able to swim and hear in a pool. I wish I had my camera because Steve was going to town splashing around like a crazy man. I had to wonder what the two ladies sitting in pool chairs thought. If you didn't know any better, you would think he was either drowning or learning how to swim. Of course, I knew better. He was listening to the water. I splashed right along with him.

It was pretty interesting to hear the water when I was under water and to hear it while I was doing the back stroke and such. The best part was being able to have a conversation in the water. The two ladies got in the pool after a while and we told them about our adventure. We would have had to read their lips before.

I decided to shower with my ear on, too, when I got home. While I was at it I decided I should sing in there, too. I sang *Singing in the Rain*. I figured that was an appropriate song for the occasion and it was how I felt, too.

June 9, 2013 Week Three Update and Walk4Hearing

It's been a little over three weeks now since I've had my new ear. I haven't had any new "wow" moments lately, but I am still amazed by it. I have been wearing mostly my new ear alone when I've been at home. The other day I forgot to take off the old ear and started doing my rehab exercises. I was shocked at how clear and easy one of the exercises was. Then I realized I was listening with *both* ears. Oops! They sure do sound great together. I had both of my ears on last night when Bob came home and I was able to understand him so clearly. He was in the kitchen and I was in the living room. I even understood what he was saying when he was muttering to himself in front of the refrigerator. It will be nice when I get the new ear up to where the old ear is so that I can wear them both together all of the time. The new ear is coming along very well, very quickly. I can definitely see progress from week to week. It's going to take longer for voices to sound more normal, but it will come.

Today was the Walk4Hearing in Long Beach. I helped out at the Advanced Bionics booth before the walk. I talked to four different people that would greatly benefit from getting implants. I hope I convinced them to get tested. I believe their lives would drastically change if they do. We had a nice 5K walk along the marina and then there was a pizza party afterwards with all of the Advanced Bionics employees. A couple of them came up to me and said they recognized me from my speech.

I have noticed that I am doing really well in noisy situations. The Advanced Bionics booth was right next to a loud speaker blaring music the whole time we were there. I was able to understand everybody with no problems. I also went to the R/C Expo where a friend of mine was inducted into the Hall of Fame. It was quite loud at the tables at the banquet but I understood everybody at our table, too, although they were having a hard time understanding *me* because it was so loud. That was a switch. I understood the majority of the speech that was given, as well as most of the people accepting awards, too.

June 17, 2013 Cambria Trip

Bob and I spent a long weekend in Cambria, California with stops in Santa Barbara and Morro Bay. We went on a tour at LotusLand in Santa Barbara. It was a two-mile, two-hour docent led tour. The docent was a seventy-plus year old Irish woman with an accent. It was a really beautiful tour and I highly recommend it. I was happy to discover that I could understand the docent when I was paying attention. Most of the time, however, I admit I wasn't really paying attention.

One of my hobbies is photography so I tended to lag behind and shoot pictures rather than staying with the group and actively listen. When I *did* listen, she was pretty fascinating. Fortunately, Bob got everything she said so I was able to ask him about the things I was unclear about later.

When we were in Cambria, we took a tour of Hearst Castle. I had a couple of "wow" moments there. Alex Trebek did the narration on the bus ride to and from the castle. I understood every word that he said. I understood probably half of what our tour guide said. I am afraid I have developed a bad habit, over the years, of not paying attention to tour guides because I normally have to stand right in front of them and concentrate too hard on reading their lips. I was amazed that I could stand anywhere in the room, even the largest rooms, and still hear her voice. It was definitely loud enough no matter where I stood. When I really paid attention, I could get a lot of what she said. Of course, if I looked at her I got all of it. I even heard the alarm beep when Bob stepped on the carpet that he wasn't supposed to.

We went to see the elephant seals. I had never seen elephant seals before. They sure looked funny. I enjoyed listening to them as they sparred in the ocean. I was surprised how loud they were. I can only imagine how loud it would be if they were mating.

We went on a really nice walk on the boardwalk at Moonstone Beach in Cambria and did some geocaching.

We went to Montana de Oro park near Morro Bay and went for a five mile hike on the Point Buchon trail. The scenery around every turn was just stunning.

I didn't do any "active" rehab exercises on the trip and I wore both ears the whole time. I noticed, today, that my new ear was hearing almost the same thing as my old ear. I decided to do some comprehension tests on both ears by themselves and together. I found that both ears, separately, are understanding almost the same things. Both ears, together, are understanding about 10% more than when they are apart. I am getting about 60% comprehension on consonant sounds and 80% comprehension on vowel sounds. I am going to try something different on my rehab now. I am going to continue to do my rehab exercises, but I will alternate ears every other day rather than only working on my new ear and see how that goes. In any case, the new ear has advanced at an astounding rate and I am very pleased with the progress.

I did have trouble in a couple of the restaurants in Cambria but I noticed that Bob was asking *me* to repeat myself just as much as I was asking him to. I guess it was more the restaurants than my hearing in those two places. I will do more rehab to help with listening in noisy environments, too.

June 27, 2013 Positive Attitude Makes a Difference

I have been asked a lot, lately, how I can always have such a positive attitude. I got my positive outlook from my mom very early on. She taught me not to dwell on things I couldn't do, or didn't have, but to focus on what I could do. We have done a great deal of traveling together and we have always had an incredibly good time. Why? Because we never worried about what anybody thought of us and we didn't worry about anything we couldn't change. We always looked to see the good things and didn't waste our time being negative. There have been plenty of negative things that have happened, however. Ironically, my mother often recalls our trips by what bad things happened on them. We joke that if something bad didn't happen, she wouldn't remember the trip. The key to a happy life, though, is not to constantly dwell on the negatives.

I will be the first to tell you that I have my bad days and complain like everybody else. Patience is definitely not something that I have a lot of. When I get too upset, though, I try to remember a great speaker I once heard, Henry Marsh, who told us that we can change how we are feeling. We have that power. If you are able to change your situation, then by all means, do so. Sometimes getting angry or upset has brought about great change. Think about laws and charities and other things that came to be because somebody got too upset. But if you aren't able to change the situation, worrying about it or getting upset about it, really isn't going to make any difference at all. It will only make you unhappy. I was reminded of that on my way home from work a couple of days ago. I knew it was going to take me forever to get home as soon as I got on the freeway. It was like a parking lot. Normally, this would make my blood boil and the road rage would set in. But then I remembered that I didn't have to be upset. I had the power to make it a positive experience. Hmmm, stop and go traffic means no road noise. Music is excellent in my car, especially with no road noise. So I put on my favorite Styx CD and listened to my heart's content. Because it was so quiet in there and I had so much time, I took the time to really listen to every instrument and really paid attention to everything I was hearing. At other times I have chosen to get off the freeway and take a different route to see some different scenery along the way. If I get off early enough I can drive down the coast. It's stop and go there, too, but it's beautiful. Sometimes, if I can't get off the freeway, I simply really look at the buildings I pass. How many times do we really *look* at what we see every single day? You might be surprised to find some interesting buildings, a business you might want to go to, cool trees, or something else that catches your eye if you really look.

I remember when I was early in on my relationship with Bob. He would get me so angry sometimes. I would sulk and cry and get depressed for a while. I noticed, however, that Bob was going about his business as he always was. My attitude seemed to have absolutely no affect on him. Then I thought how stupid was I? I was the one who was making myself unhappy and yet, he was the one that was "wrong". Isn't the other person always the one who is wrong? I realized I had the power to change my attitude, and I did. I asked him later why he wasn't upset and he said he knew I would get over it. He just had to wait long enough. Smart man, that Bob!

Sometimes success or failure can simply be a matter of how you view a situation. I had the ladies over for Stamp Night last night. I was busy stamping away and wasn't really paying too much attention to the conversations so I didn't understand the conversations going on around me. But at one point, one of my customers asked me a question and I knew exactly who was talking to me. I'd call that a success. If you keep your expectations small and appreciate the little things, you will have a lot of successes in your life.

When people are just getting their implant turned on, I recommend that they keep a daily journal of what they are hearing. It's important to write down the new sounds no matter how minor they may seem. That way, when they get discouraged about the big picture not coming fast enough, they can look back and see how much all of those little things add up. They can also write down issues they are having problems with. It helps their audiologist fix those problems and, oftentimes, those problems disappear after a little while and that, too, helps them see how far they have come.

Here's a challenge for you: every day for the next seven days, find something positive in your day. It can be something as simple as enjoying the flowers in your neighborhood or listening to the birds sing. Find something good in someone else and give them a compliment. Not only will it make you feel good, it will make them feel great. When is the last time you thanked your spouse for making a great meal? When is the last time you told your significant other how "hot" they are? When is the last time you've admired something someone was wearing and told them? Try it!

July 2, 2013 My Take on CI Rehab

I look at my CI surgery in the same way as my mom's knee replacement surgery. When she got out of the hospital, she was not able to ride a bike. Instead, they sent her home with a walker and she had to exercise, at home, for thirty minutes three times a day. She also had to walk around the house for five minutes every hour. She did that for a few weeks and then she went to the doctor's office and did physical therapy there for an hour, three times a week. She did that for many weeks. It was pretty intense at physical therapy. She worked out on lots of machines. She eventually ditched the walker and started using a cane. Then she got rid of the cane and walked on her own. She was even able to pedal a bike at PT. She heard from several people that quit doing therapy too early that their knees became stiff. I have no doubt that if she didn't do the therapy at all that she would still be using that walker.

Getting a CI is like that. Think of your hearing aid or other ear as using crutches. You *have* to retrain the brain how to use that CI. Your brain is going to take the easy way out and go with what is familiar, ie: listening to the hearing aid or other ear, just as it has done before. It is very important that you exercise your CI ear by itself without using the crutches, at the very least while you are doing your rehab exercises. I highly recommend that you spend an hour a day doing "active" rehab exercises. But you also need to "walk around the house every hour" by "passively" listening. For example, keep a radio or TV on. Take your crutches off while you do that, too. You do not have to do the sixty minutes of active listening all at one time. You can do each exercise at different times throughout the day if you want to. The key is to *do* them and do them without hearing anything in the other ear. Ditch the crutches.

Start off slowly doing the exercises the easy way just like my mom did at home. Read along using the scripts on the audio and phone exercises. There is no shame in that. Then listen without the scripts and see how much you are able to understand. Try to read and listening along with an audiobook for thirty minutes a day. Start with children's books that you can easily follow along with before moving up to John Grisham novels or whoever your favorite author is. Listen to newscasts on TV, as they are the easiest to understand. Then work your way up to your favorite shows. Use the closed captioning. Eventually, you won't need to.

Nobody said this was going to be easy. My mom was not a happy camper while she did those exercises. I'll tell you one thing though, I much prefer listening to an audiobook that I enjoy and watching TV with my CI alone any day over doing the physical exercises that she had to do. We have it easy that's for sure.

I have a daily rehab group on Facebook. I post four exercises a day there, including phone, audio, Angel Sound and an "other" exercise. If you have a CI and would like to join us, search Cochlear Implant Daily Rehab.

July 7, 2013 Kayaking

I went kayaking yesterday with a couple of friends. That wasn't a new adventure. I have been kayaking before. What *was* new was that I was able to hear while we went around the harbor. You don't take the chance of falling into the water wearing expensive hearing aids so I never wore them while kayaking. But yesterday, I put on the waterproof configuration on my Neptune processor and I got to hear everything. It was great!

July 11, 2013 Test Time

I went in for speech tests today. I have written about this subject before. See December 11, 2012 "Second Mapping / First Test" for more detailed information than what I am going to say here.

My left ear has been activated for almost two months now. We did the AZBio Sentence Test, which is where I hear a variety of sentences read by several different people. I got 84% and 92% on that test using just my new ear. One of the voices had a munchkin sounding woman. I did the worst when she spoke. With both ears, I got 94% and 91%. It was just astonishing, especially when you consider I got 0% with my hearing aids. Yes, you read that right.

We also did a CNC Word Test. These are random words. Using only my new ear, I got 74% on words and 89% with phonemes. Phonemes means I said a word that sounded like the right word. For example, I said "height" and it was "hike". With both ears I got 76% on words and 85% on phonemes. When I was tested at one month with my right ear, I only got 38% and 4% with my hearing aids so this is a pretty dramatic improvement.

July 29, 2013 Stampin' Up! Convention

I have been a Stampin' Up! Demonstrator for twenty years. Every year Stampin' Up! has a convention in Salt Lake City for its demonstrators. Usually there are about 3,000 people that attend. This year was the largest one yet with 5,800 people there. It is the company's twenty-fifth anniversary so it was a big one.

Stampin' Up! is really great in accommodating demonstrators with special needs. They have a front row reserved for blind and hard of hearing/deaf demonstrators and a friend. I have sat there for many years and I have been able to meet some phenomenal hearing-impaired stampers. Two of these women, Becky Roberts and Diana Gibbs, are in the top one hundred in the whole company and that is saying a *lot* since there are probably forty thousand active demonstrators if not more. Becky's hearing loss is pretty profound, so it truly is miraculous what she has been able to do with her business.

This was my first convention with my cochlear implants and I was anxious to see what I could and couldn't do. As in all cases such as this, I tried very hard to keep my expectations very low so that I wouldn't be disappointed. In fact, I was almost dreading the general sessions as I thought they might be too loud and overwhelming. They have presentations on the main stage for *all* 5,800 of us at one time. That's a *lot* of very excited women in one room. Believe me when they tell us we are all getting free stamps that the crowd goes wild.

I noticed a difference in the presentations immediately. They have big screens on the side but they don't always show the presenters on the screens. I usually have to either read their lips or turn around and read the teleprompter to understand what they are saying. Oftentimes, I have missed the majority of what guest speakers have said because they did not use the teleprompter. It is very frustrating and quite frankly, lonely, to have an entire audience laughing when you can't understand anything. This time I understood the CEO clearly but I could do that with my hearing aids. She has a great voice. But then they showed a video with no captions. It was an interview with three people talking. I could easily understand two of the people but missed a lot of what the third one said, but hey, I'll take it. I never would have understood any of it with hearing aids. They showed several videos over the three days and I was amazed that I understood the majority of what was said, even with voiceovers. While I was thrilled for myself, I looked at Becky sitting next to me texting away, realizing that she was not getting any of it. That was me just last year. I felt so bad for her and wished she could experience what I was experiencing.

Throughout the convention there were many different presenters in different rooms. Again, normally, I would sit in the front of each of these rooms but this time I decided to move around, just to see what I could understand. At one class I sat towards the back. It was too far back to read lips. I understood the presenter well. Well enough to know that we should ditch the class because it was too basic for us. At another class, I didn't understand hardly anything. The sound was echoing all over the room and the presenter's voice was not in a good range for me. Fortunately, that wasn't a class I really needed to understand but it was good practice for me. We sat in the middle of the giant room for another presentation and I understood the three different presenters really well. We sat at the very back of the closing general session because we had to get out of there as soon as it ended to catch our plane and I was just so amazed that I was able to understand so much of it.

Oftentimes, there are product demonstrations and that is what they show on the screens, not the speaker's face. Normally, I have to choose: read lips and miss the stamping demonstration or watch the screen and not understand what they are saying. Not this time. I was able to watch the big screen *and* understand what they were saying while they were stamping. It was fantastic!

The crowds were *not* too loud at all. And when it was really loud, my friends could easily yell into my ear and I understood what they were saying. In the past I would have to read their lips and not actually hear them.

I think my biggest "wow" moment of the whole convention came during the twenty-fifth anniversary party one night. All 5,800 of us were in a giant room all spread out. There was an 80's band playing, acrobatics doing their performance from the ceiling, desserts galore, carnival type games, trivia, bingo, and more. I spotted some hip hop dancers when we came in so, after checking everything out, I decided to go and watch the dancers. I knew I wouldn't be able to make out what the band was playing, and knew I wouldn't be able to hear anything but drums, but I could easily watch the dancers. But wait a minute. That was the *old* Julie. I used to have to have people tell me what songs were playing and maybe I would finally catch on halfway through after watching people dance and reading lips. I could feel the vibrations and could hear beats, but it was usually too loud and I wasn't able to really get it. Imagine how surprised I was when I went over to the dance floor and actually knew what songs the band was singing just by listening. I just couldn't believe it! I heard all of the instruments and I could easily figure out each song that was being played right from the start. It wasn't long before I got out there on the dance floor and danced the night away and sang along to every song. I stayed until the very last song played and danced the entire time. I was in heaven.

The convention itself was fantastic, especially since it was the twenty-fifth anniversary, but it was a convention that I am sure I won't soon forget just because I was finally able to be almost like everybody else. Miracles really do happen!

August 2, 2013 # Styx Concert

I debated on whether or not I should write about this. As you may have guessed, I try to be positive but this is a book about my hearing journey and, therefore, I think it needs to be realistic, too. That means that some experiences are not always going to be positive. This is one of them.

Styx is probably my favorite band of all time. I went to see their concert when I was a kid and I have been as an adult. The last time I saw them was about four years ago at the House of Blues. A friend of mine had an extra ticket to tonight's Styx concert and asked if I wanted to go. I had actually been debating about buying my own ticket to the concert for about a month. Was I really ready to face what I would hear? I wasn't so sure, and I didn't get my own ticket.

I went to the concert with realistic expectations. I expected the instruments to sound really good and the vocals to sound pretty bad. My wish was that I would be able to understand what they said between songs. My fantasy was that Dennis DeYoung would rejoin the band. He was one of the original members who left the band long ago.

Music with the CI has been a major readjustment for me. Here are a couple of things for you to think about. Imagine if you lost your loved one and all of the pictures of them have been replaced with someone else in the pictures. How long would it take for you to forget what your loved one looked like? Now imagine that you go to bed tonight and when you wake up tomorrow, every vocal in every record you have ever known has been replaced by a handful of bands that sound nothing like the original singers. The songs are the same ones you've loved for years and the instruments are all the same, but you may never hear the original singers ever again. No more Styx, no more Elton John, no more Michael Jackson, no more Rolling Stones, no more Carrie Underwood, no more (fill in the blank with your favorite singers here). All you have left is your memory of what they sounded like. Sure, you can play their records, but remember, it isn't their voice singing on them anymore, someone else is.

Now, I have been listening to music like that since I got my CI and I have done a pretty good job of accepting that . . . until tonight. Tonight it kind of hit me like a ton of bricks that I may never hear Styx the way I remember them ever again in my lifetime. What if I forget how they sound? That thought terrifies and saddens me. Man, I sure hope that I am wrong. I know that Advanced Bionics is working on new technology all the time. I am still relatively new to this CI game and my ears and brain are still adapting. I know that some people have done really well with music and they do remember music the way that it used to be. That gives me hope. But for now, for lack of better words . . . it sucks!

The concert was bittersweet for me. The songs were still some of my favorite songs of all time and I got a lot out of it but it may as well just been some random band singing the songs because it wasn't Styx. In a way, it actually made me happy that it wasn't Dennis DeYoung singing because nobody else got to hear the real guy either. They did get to hear Tommy Shaw, though, and the Dennis replacement does sound a lot like Dennis (from what I remember a few years ago) so it's not the same as what I was hearing.

I tried to explain what I was hearing and feeling to my friend after the concert but she really can't grasp the enormity of it. She said that I just need to accept the new reality and she is right. That is what I have been doing. But sometimes you just want to see your loved one's face again and you want to hear your favorite song the way you remember it one more time.

At one point in the concert the band was taking a break except for the "new" Dennis. He was getting the crowd to sing along to bits and pieces of popular non-Styx songs. At one point he sang the Rolling Stones' "You can't always get what you want. You can't always get what you want. You can't always get what you want. But if you try, sometimes you just might find, you get what you need." I couldn't help but think he was talking to me. I do need the CI. It has been a real blessing in my life and I don't, for a second, regret getting it. If I had to do it again, I would do it in a minute.

Oh, and by the way, my wish came true. I *did* understand everything they said between songs. It was awesome!

August 4, 2013 Air Combat Fighter Jet Experience

I went to the Flightdeck Air Combat Center in Anaheim a while ago to go on the Boeing 737 Flight Simulator. While I was doing that, I saw something that looked like it would be a lot more fun: the Fox-1 Mission Fighter Jet Experience. At the time I did the Boeing flight, I was still wearing hearing aids. I saw that they were wearing headphones and knew I couldn't do that. The microphone on my hearing aids were on top of my ear and, besides not being able to wear the headphones in the proper placement, I knew it wouldn't be loud enough either. But it sure looked like those guys were having fun.

After I got my first CI, the fighter jet experience came up on Groupon so I bought it. I decided to wait until I had my second CI to use it. Well . . . it was awesome. We had to sit through a class to learn how to fly the plane, how to shoot the other planes down, and which button to push to trash talk the other pilots. I was a little worried when the instructor started talking because he had a really deep voice, but it turned out to be no problem. I understood everything he said and I made sure to know how close I needed to be to push the "kill" button. Ha!

Then we all suited up and went to the simulators. There was a giant screen in front of us. We were to fly the not-so-friendly skies and kill or be killed. I put on my headphone and was pleased that it was comfortable on my ear. My CI T-Mic microphone sits at the entrance of my ear canal so I can wear it normally. Then came the precheck of all of the pilots. I heard him clearly as he said, "307, do you copy?" "Copy" I replied. Then we all took off. Uh, this sure sounded a lot easier in the class. I guess I was all over the place because one of the instructors came and gave me private lessons. Evidently, I was doing too many barrel rolls. Well, they *are* fun.

Then it was time to get down to business. I had several other planes in my sight and made my first kill. Yes! Unfortunately, after I made each kill I somehow managed to fly off into oblivion at 20,000 feet and had a heck of a time finding anybody again. I did manage to make four kills and only got killed four times. Once was of my own doing and a couple times because they had to kill me because I had flown too far away.

Then we had four chances to land the plane. I swam with the fishes three times and crashed onto the airstrip once. I noticed the guy next to me was also swimming with me so that made me happy. I also noticed he was laughing just as hard as I was.

My brother, Curtis, once told me that I was not a "real" girl. I guess he was right. There were a lot of women there but I was the only one that flew with the men. The other ladies sat and watched. It's not unusual for me to be the only woman doing the "guy stuff" like racing race cars or go carts. Why is that, ladies? The guys do it because it's *fun*. You should join them. If somebody gave me $200 and told me to race a car or go shopping, I'd race the car every time.

Speaking of racing cars, before my CI, I went to do the Mario Andretti Racing Experience. I was supposed to drive a Formula One car. Unfortunately, because I couldn't wear the headphones, I had to do a ride along instead. That was still a lot of fun because we went a heck of a lot faster than the students did, but it would still be fun to do it myself. I think I could probably do it now.

August 18, 2013 Crazy Dreams and Residual Hearing

Boy, I sure had some crazy dreams last night. In the first one, I lay in bed with my back to Bob. He started talking to me and I heard him. That was a miracle, so I asked him to whisper and I heard him then, too. Evidently, my residual hearing had been retained and, even better than that, my hearing had been restored. Then I dreamed of seeing a demonstration where they stamped on t-shirts and made these really cool designs. Then it switched to my cousin, Sue, telling me that she had a boyfriend. Then she explained that she didn't really have a boyfriend, but she was going to tell her friend's mother she did because her friend's mom was trying to fix her up with her son and she wasn't interested. Then I dreamt that I found this cute blue and red bird in my house. I caught him and trapped him under a very small plastic bag. That one had multiple endings: the bird died; I let him go in the yard; I took him to my cousin, Susan, who rehabilitates birds; I took him to another cousin, Leroy, who is crazy about birds; and I took him to Petco. I also dreamt I found a geocache in a park that had coordinates written on a toothpick that took geocachers more than three hours to find. Oh wait, that one was true. Crazy!

But let's go back to the one on residual hearing. First of all, before I got my CI, my residual hearing was pretty much non-existent. The only way I could hear Bob without wearing my hearing aids was if he spoke directly into my ear and even that was iffy. Now that I have CIs, my residual hearing is gone. It was lost during surgery and I am completely 100% deaf, which I knew ahead of time and fully accepted.

Since I had my surgery, Advanced Bionics has released a new electrode that they are implanting in people now. It's called the Mid-Scala electrode. That electrode *does* retain peoples' residual hearing. I did know about it, and could have waited for it, but I didn't know how long the FDA was going to take to approve it. I knew I really didn't have any residual hearing worth saving so I decided not to wait. I was told that the technology (what I would hear with my processor) was the same in both electrodes and that was the important part to me. It turns out the new electrode came out just a couple of months after my second surgery. They are implanting people with that one now, but I have no regrets on not waiting.

When I'm in bed I don't have my CI on which means that I am completely deaf. So how do Bob and I communicate in bed? Bob "writes" on my back, stomach, leg — wherever. It's actually quite comical because I have to ask him where the top of the letters are so I know which direction he is writing as it's usually sideways. Add the fact that he writes his letters in a different way than I write mine and it can take quite some time for me to figure out what he is trying to tell me. He'll rub on my back to "erase" what he wrote and tap on my back to tell me I got it right.

So why don't we just use sign language? I wanted both of us to take sign language a long time ago, but he didn't want to. He gets quite a kick out of talking to me using his "writing on my body" method. Besides, if it's dark you can't see sign language anyway. I didn't take the class by myself because it's like taking French. Learning French isn't worth much if you don't know anybody else that speaks French. I did learn how to finger spell when I was a kid and I still know how to do that, except for a couple of letters. I also know the signs for "yes" and "no", although I get them mixed up. I know the sign for "bathroom" and "eat" too. I learned those when my brother, Steve, taught his son, Joel, some words when he was a baby before he learned how to talk.

The only thing I figured I would miss when I lost my residual hearing was the ability to hear myself. I even asked my surgeon about this. I think he thought I was nuts. I have always been able to hear myself speak without my hearing aids on. How is that possible if I can't hear anyone else? Fortunately, even with CIs, I can still hear myself speak. I realized I wasn't crazy when another person that I was mentoring asked me that same question. We have the same surgeon and, apparently, he thought she was nuts, too. It must have something to do with vibrations or maybe it's just our brain filling in what it knows we are saying and knows what we sound like. Whatever the reason, I'm really happy about that.

August 24, 2013 At the Office

We recently moved our offices. I am now in a large office with no walls. I have a row of file cabinets separating me and the lady next to me, Lorna. Then there is another desk on the opposite side of her where Annie sits. Next to Annie is Pete. Pete has a partition in front of him. If I am sitting at my desk, I can't see any of them.

With hearing aids, I would have to look at the person speaking to be able to read their lips. I definitely couldn't understand what somebody was saying outside my office. Lorna usually talks pretty loudly when she talks to me. It's probably why we have gotten along so well over the many years we have worked together. I could always understand her. Yesterday, she was having a quieter conversation with Annie. I could easily understand what both of them were saying and jumped into the conversation. I noticed Lorna's volume went up when she realized I was listening. It's just a habit, I guess. I was pretty amazed that I was able to keep working and hear, and participate in the conversation, too.

Sometimes I have a quick question for Pete who's way at the opposite end of the room. I can now easily simply ask him the question and get my answer. No more having to go over to his desk or shoot him an email to wait for an answer. Sometimes he yells his answer back and I tell him that he doesn't have to do that. He can simply answer in his normal voice.

I used to not be able to use my office phone. Now, not only can I use it, I can also use either ear to listen to it. That's strange. Even in the olden days when I could use the phone, I only used my left ear. I couldn't hear as well out of the right ear.

At one point in the day, Lorna came up to my desk and she was crying. I couldn't understand why. I didn't see anybody upset her. Then she said, "You answered me!" Evidently, I had said "thank you" or "you're welcome" or something little like that. What she couldn't believe is that the vacuum cleaner was going and I still was able to understand what she said and commented on it. I'm used to crying at my "wow" moments but not used to other people having that reaction. I guess I'm taking these "wow" moments for granted because I didn't even think twice about it.

I can also tell who is coming down the hall without seeing them. One girl drags her feet and I can hear another girl's flip flops. I can also hear the break bell and the forklift in the warehouse far away.

September 15, 2013 First Bionic Ear Association Gathering

I am a volunteer mentor for the Bionic Ear Association (BEA). The BEA is a support group from Advanced Bionics (AB) which is the company I got my cochlear implant from. There are many chapters of the BEA but they didn't have one in Orange County, California where I live. I was asked to be the Chapter Leader. I asked what that entailed. I was told that they like to have events where people with cochlear implants can come and meet each other, and people that are thinking about getting one can learn more about them.

I have seen pictures of the gatherings they have in San Francisco and they have some pretty incredible food spreads there. Anybody that knows me knows that I live on TV dinners and definitely don't cook so I was a little hesitant to accept. I didn't want to kill anybody at our first event. But I was assured that we could cater and just have deli sandwiches and cookies. I was pretty relieved about that. I accepted and now I am the Chapter Leader of the new Orange County Chapter of the BEA.

We picked the date for our first gathering. My first task was to find a location. I thought about different restaurants but they all were going to be too noisy. Then I remembered the clubhouse in my neighborhood. It seemed to be the right size and there was an outdoor area in case people wanted a quiet place to chat. Unfortunately, I hadn't gone inside. I didn't realize that the acoustics were really noisy and had quite an echo until we had already given everyone the location. Fortunately, this group is *very* good at reading lips. To my surprise, we had forty-five people signed up to come. Not bad for a first event.

I have been working with my rep from AB, Sarah Hargest, to make the event a success. I came up with the idea to have a "Wishes and Wows" segment as part of the presentation we were doing. I asked people who were thinking about getting a CI to dare to dream and to make up a wish list of all of the things they hoped to hear some day. I asked the people that already had a CI to make up a list of their "wow" moments, which are those things they could do now that they couldn't do before they had a CI. I also asked the hearing guests that came with them to make up similar lists.

We started the day with lunch. We had six tables. I made sure to sit someone with a CI at each table. I matched people up ahead of time that I thought would hit it off. Maybe they had the same hearing history or were the same age, for example. Some of the people I had been mentoring, some I had already had the privilege of meeting in person, and some I had gotten to know on Facebook or in forums. It was really neat to be able to have them meet each other for the first time.

I had also made up a "Getting to Know You" game where I had various statements like "I am fluent in sign language", "I had surgery last month", etc. They were to go around the room and find the people that matched those statements. That was supposed to happen in the first hour. We wound up not doing the game because everyone was having such great conversations during lunch. That was a good thing.

The second hour was our presentation. I gave a short talk on my experience leading up to getting my CI. I knew that the things I went through were likely the same for most of the people that were there and that they would be able to relate. I really wanted to emphasize our common bond and that they weren't alone in their experiences. I realize, now, that it was probably really good for the hearing people to hear that speech as they might not have realized some of the things their loved ones went through. Then I went around to each person and asked them to tell us just one of their wishes and wows. I was very pleased that every person participated. Their answers really moved me. So many of their wishes were the same wishes I had before I got my CI, and all of their wishes have turned into wows for me so far. I kept wanting to say, "Yes! That will happen for you!" but I didn't. Well, maybe a couple of times I did. I just couldn't resist. I am really hoping that in six months those people will have had their CI and will be able to say that their wishes came true. I think the wows that people shared really encouraged people, too.

Then Sarah gave a really great presentation on the new Naida CI Q70 processor that was just released. I just got mine. See the next chapter for my experience with that. She was very good and I know people really appreciated hearing her information. I even got to model some of the things she was talking about. Move over, Heidi Klum.

The last hour was spent mingling with the guests. They also got to go to the Advanced Bionics table where they could try on the new processor and pick up literature about it. Most importantly, they got to talk to Sarah and a couple of the other AB reps and ask them questions. People were also able to ask me questions during that time. It was really great to see so many people conversing with each other. I think a lot of long lasting friendships were formed. I got to talk to many of the people as they left, too, which I thoroughly enjoyed.

You may have been wondering how my brother, Steve, has been doing with his CI. Okay, I'm getting choked up now. Hold on! When I first told Steve that we were going to have this gathering, he told me I was crazy. He said that we would never understand each other. I pointed out to him that this was exactly why we were having it. We could finally meet people who were just like us. None of us were going to be able to hear very well so it was perfectly okay to ask people to repeat themselves. We would *all* "get it." I also pointed out that, because he has a CI, that he (probably for the first time in his life) would actually be one of the people that would hear and understand *better* than many of the people that were going to be there. He was pretty excited to go after that.

Since Steve has a CI, I sat him at a table with people that I thought would benefit from meeting him. One was a friend that he met at his church that has a profound hearing loss. One was a lady that wanted to know more about Kaiser (they would be sharing the same doctor and audiologist). One had the same hearing history that he did. I thought it was valuable that he share his experience with her. Every time I saw Steve he was talking to someone else. (Okay, full out crying now. I'm such a sap.) I knew he was doing okay. It was so great to see him being so social. I can't remember when I've seen him like that before. He seemed to be smiling every time I looked at him. I also knew how many people he was helping. I was truly grateful to him for putting himself out there to help those people. I know they got a lot out of their conversations with him. He also told me that he didn't need to read the captions during the presentations and that he had no problems in the noisy room (and yes, it *was* too noisy). I am *so* happy for him.

All in all it was a great success. We achieved everything we set out to and more. We are definitely going to need a bigger place for the next one (and a quieter place, too) because I have a feeling a lot of people will be back. I am sure Steve is looking forward to our next one and I know I am, too.

September 19, 2013 New Naida CI Q70 Processor Review

Advanced Bionics finally got FDA approval of the new Naida CI Q70 behind the ear (BTE) processor. I am fortunate that my insurance gives me two processors per ear so I was able to get them. First off, you pronounce

Naida (nah-EE-duh). I've had it for a almost a week now and this is going to be a fairly long, detailed, review as there is a lot to cover.

As soon as the FDA approved it, I got an email from Advanced Bionics saying that I could order it. They sent me an order form and a link to where to order it online. Sounds easy, right? Not! Man, there are a lot of choices. One of the biggest ones was what color to choose. They range from blending colors like "Sand Beige" and "Silver Gray" to wild colors like "Dragon Orange" and "Electric Green." They have a neat "Alpine White" that makes it look like a Bluetooth from Apple. I had been debating for some time on going with boring beige or the cool white. I definitely didn't consider a color. I have had beige hearing aids for thirty years. Who are we kidding, really? If somebody has short hair, you can easily spot a hearing aid behind their ear. When I was a teenager and in my twenties, I was self-conscious and tried to hide them, but now I could care less. So I was pretty much set on the white until a friend, Erin, said she was getting the Electric Green. I *really* liked the Caribbean Pirate. It's such a beautiful blue. It looks like the Caribbean sea. I was worried that it would clash with my clothes. Erin reminded me that I have long hair and nobody but me would really see it. She also reminded me that I have the Neptune and, if I really needed a conservative color, I could wear that. Someone else told me that I should go with the color that makes me the happiest. Well, doggone it, I'm going for the Caribbean Pirate. I'll see it every day when I put it on and take it off and they were right. It *does* make me happy. The program buttons are white on it so I went with white cables and a white headpiece. They likely will come out with a matching headpiece color later but it's not out yet. I have since seen the "boring" Sand Beige color in person and I have to say, it's anything but boring. It's actually really pretty. It has a metallic sheen to it and it's not flesh colored like so many hearing aids are.

The next big decision to make was which batteries to choose. There are three different sizes available now, with a fourth option in the works. I got three batteries per ear with any combination of these to choose from: rechargeable large PowerCel 230, rechargeable small PowerCel 110, and Zinc-Air Battery Pak. The large ones would last all day and night, so I would not have to change them during the day. The small ones, set for my programs, last 13 1/2 hours. I would need to keep an extra set in my pocket to change them. The Zinc-Air Battery Pak holds disposable batteries that last up to 30 hours. I knew I would want one of the Zinc-Air Battery Paks (per ear) for emergency situations and for traveling in case I couldn't get to a charger easily. Some large hearing aids and even large earrings give me big headaches. I was concerned that might happen with the large batteries. However, I figured I could easily wear them for a few hours. I got one large, one small, and one Zinc-Air per ear. I will give you a review on how they fared later.

The last decision in ordering was whether to get the Phonak ComPilot, the AB myPilot remote control, the AAA PowerPak Accessory, or the Extended Battery Option. Because I have two CIs, I could choose two accessories and, fortunately, I would only need one of each option (i.e., I don't need two ComPilots). The Phonak ComPilot is very cool. It is worn around the neck and it is a Bluetooth device that allows streaming to both ears when talking on the phone, listening to music or other audio on devices like an iPhone or iPad, TV (using an extra device that's hooked up to the TV) and more. You can also use it as a remote to change programs and volume. I knew I definitely wanted the ComPilot.

I figured I wouldn't use the myPilot remote very much. It allows you to change programs and volume, change sensitivity, check your battery life, and pick the side you want to use for ZoomControl (more on that later). I used to have a remote with my hearing aids and that's just one more thing to carry around. I can easily change programs, volume, and ZoomControl simply by touching the buttons on my processor. I charge the battery every day and I can tell when the batteries are low because there is a beep that sounds every fifteen minutes for an hour before the batteries go out. I haven't had to change the sensitivity on the Neptune so I knew I didn't need that. Also, the myPilot is not always in sync with the processor. If you lock it so that it won't accidentally change programs when it's in your purse, for example, then you have to unlock it and sync it to see what program you are on. That's too much trouble for me. So who should consider getting it? Parents whose children have a CI would be a good choice. They could monitor the programs, volume, battery life, and change the programs for their children. It's ideal for them.

The AAA PowerPak is an off the ear pack that uses more than one AAA battery. I think it takes three, but don't quote me on that as it could be two.

This option has about 129 hours of charge. This would be a great option for people that go camping a lot or are away from power sources for any length of time. Personally, I would never use it so it was easy eliminating that option.

That left the Extended Battery Option. This option allowed for two extra batteries (per ear). I chose this option. Advanced Bionics is really good about allowing us to exchange unopened product for something different. I chose more of the small size batteries.

I placed my order on a Friday and this gigantic box arrived on Wednesday. I opened it up and there were two *very* nice backpacks that held all of my new goodies. I immediately fell in love with the Caribbean Pirate color. I took out my cool battery charger and started charging my batteries. I also started charging my ComPilot. That night I put everything on my processors and tried them on. They needed to be programmed so I couldn't actually use them, but I could play with them at least. The battery charger is really nice. You can charge four batteries independently and they only take a few hours to charge, as opposed to the twelve hours it took to charge my Neptune batteries.

The next day I went to my audiologist, Cheryl Tanita at Shohet Ear Associates, and got them programmed. Advanced Bionics had a webinar for the mentors so I knew how I wanted my programs to be. This part is going to be a little technical, but people with CIs will want to know this information, so here goes. My old Neptunes had three programs on them. I had ClearVoice Medium on all three programs. ClearVoice is a feature that blocks out constant background noise. My other programs had IDR 60 (for noisy places like restaurants), IDR 70 (everyday program) and IDR 80 (for music). IDR stands for Input Dynamic Range. IDR allows for how much sound we can hear. Lower numbers let in less sound and higher numbers let in more sound. The Naida has five program slots. Sounds great, however, there are more features and those features require their own slots. I was actually going to have to give up some of my old programs. I knew I needed to keep IDR 70 and I used IDR 60 more than IDR 80 so I decided to forgo the IDR 80 program. I would still have my Neptunes and could use that program on there if I needed to. This is what I decided my new programs would be:

Program 1) IDR 70, CV Medium (my old every day program)

Program 2) IDR 70, CV Medium + new UltraZoom feature

Program 3) IDR 70, CV Medium + new DuoPhone feature

Program 4) IDR 70, CV Medium + new ZoomControl feature

Program 5) IDR 60 + new UltraZoom feature

100% T-Mic, 75% ComPilot on all programs. QuickSync, Optima, and alerts turned on.

Now it was time to get out in the real world. When I left Cheryl, I wore a small battery on one ear and a large battery on the other ear. I wanted to see if I could feel the difference. I couldn't. In fact, the whole processor is so light and comfortable I really couldn't feel them at all. It didn't seem like I was wearing anything. Awesome! It is so nice not to have the long cables from the Neptune or have the Neptune processor clipped to my belt. There are no more goofy bulges. I will continue to use the Neptune for watersports and when I get out of the shower with wet hair but that will probably be all. The DuoPhone feature allows you to hold up a phone to one ear and the voices stream to the opposite ear, too. I tried that out but it didn't seem to work. I'm assuming my audiologist probably didn't program it right. I go back next month and I'll have her check it then. I went out to dinner that night with my family and used program two with IDR 70, CV Medium and the new UltraZoom program. The UltraZoom feature allows the sound in front of you to come in loud and clear while the sounds to the side and behind are lowered. I did seem to hear better at the restaurant, however, it was a fairly quiet restaurant.

The next day I decided to wear the large batteries all day, but put the small batteries in my pocket just in case the large batteries bothered me later. This would be my first full day with the new processor. I went to the office that day and it went well. I used the ComPilot and listened to music with it. It's *great*. With the Neptunes, I plugged a cord from my iPhone into my Neptune and the sound would go to one ear. With the ComPilot, I put it around my neck and didn't plug anything in anywhere. It is wireless and the Bluetooth streamed the music to both ears. I was also able to leave my phone on my desk and move freely around the office and the music still played on. I'm not sure what my co-workers think of my dancing at the copy machine but they'll get used to it. I drove my car on my way home from work. It does not have any Bluetooth capabilities so I haven't used my phone in the car. Not now. I took out the ComPilot, put it around my neck and had a thirty minute phone conversation. The ComPilot works the way that DuoPhone is supposed to. It streams the voice on the phone to both ears. However, you do not have to hold the phone up to your ear like you do with DuoPhone. It's hands free. It worked beautifully. I understood probably 99% of the conversation. Excellent!

That night was Friday the 13th and I went on a ninety minute guided Ghost Tour with three of my friends in Orange. I have to interject here and say that if I still had my hearing aids, I would *never* have gone on this tour. I would have had to stand directly in front of the tour guide and would have had to read her lips for ninety minutes. Add the fact that it was dark outside and she would be in shadows. There's no way I would have enjoyed myself. The CI, however, allowed me to understand everything she said. She even had one of those headset microphones that went directly in front of her lips. I wouldn't have been able to read her lips if I tried. She was also in the dark sometimes but I understood her clearly. I also didn't have to stand right in front of her, which came in handy when she got a little boring and I let my mind wander. My being able to understand her was not a result of the Naida's features but a result of having a CI. By about 8:30 pm, my right ear was bothering me. The weight from the large batteries was felt at that point. I changed to my smaller battery. The left ear was fine.

The ZoomControl feature works similar to the UltraZoom feature. But the UltraZoom feature allows you to hear what is straight ahead of you, and the ZoomControl allows you to hear from either the right side or the left side. When you push the program button on the processor on the side that you want to hear, it transmits the sound from that side to the other side and blocks out the noise that is really coming from the other side. The whole group was walking from one house to another. I was having a hard time hearing my friend, Doris, because of all of the chatter going on around us. I remembered the ZoomControl feature and decided to try it. Unfortunately, I did *not* remember that I had to push the button on the side I wanted it to work on. Doris was on my right side but I pushed the button on my left ear. Well . . . it worked. All too well, I'm afraid. Because I pushed the button on my left side, I couldn't hear Doris at all. Oops! By the time I realized what I had done we were at the next house and I had to switch back to the first program. I probably should have tried it in the car but there were three of us in there and I was in the backseat and I wanted to hear what the people in the front seat were saying, so I didn't. By the way, I understood about half of what the driver was saying and everything the person next to me and the person in the back seat said. I couldn't have done that with hearing aids, especially at night. I haven't used the ZoomControl since then so the jury is still out on that one, but it does appear that it was programmed properly. I can see that this would be great to use on long drives and on Porsche rallies.

Saturday was a big Bionic Ear Association social (see the last chapter). I didn't know how I was going to be able to hear anything due to the acoustics at the clubhouse. I sat down at my table and switched to program two (IDR 70, CV Medium, UltraZoom) but it was still a little loud. So I switched to program five (IDR 60, CV Medium, UltraZoom). Wow! What a difference. It was really great. I could easily understand the people at my table. The echo from the clubhouse was gone and the noise going on all around me was greatly lowered. Every now and then I would take my processor off to show it to people. When I put it back on it automatically defaults to program one. I could immediately tell a difference and zipped right back to program five. I was very grateful to have the Naida and I knew the people that had CIs with Clear Voice were likely doing okay. My brother, Steve, did quite well there with his CI. I knew the people with just hearing aids were probably having a devil of a time but, fortunately, they are very good at reading lips.

The next day, Sunday, was another challenge. My dad, Gene Husting, used to be a co-owner of Team Associated, an R/C car company. There is a fantastic R/C museum that has opened up and they had their second "legends" day. My dad is a legend. The second I walked in the door I immediately switched to program five. The music was extremely loud there. I did fairly well at the party. Some people had voices that were just too hard to understand but others I could understand quite well. So well, in fact, that they had a harder time hearing me. That's a switch. Again, I was grateful for the new UltraZoom feature.

I no longer have any problems with the large batteries. I think my ears are used to them now and they are quite comfortable. It is very nice not having to change my batteries anymore. I had to change them at the ten-to-twelve hour mark with the Neptunes. I only have two complaints and they are very minor.

The QuickSync feature allows me to change the programs or volume on one ear and it will automatically change the programs and volume on the other ear at the same time. This is a nice feature. However, when the programs are changing, the processor's sound is off and I can't hear anything at all. If the change is to one program it takes probably three seconds. However, if the change is to the fifth program it can take about six seconds. That might not seem like a lot but if I'm listening to someone, I don't want to have to stop the conversation to change the program. That means I have to rely on my lipreading while the programs change. With the Neptunes, I changed one ear and then I changed the other ear so I was able to continue to hear the conversation during program changes. I can have the QuickSync turned off and may look into doing that.

All in all, the large batteries, battery charger, color, size, UltraZoom and the ComPilot are all fantastic. The jury is still out on DuoPhone and ZoomControl but I'm looking forward to using them.

October 1, 2013 The New Normal

I was reflecting back on the last week and realized that I had many new "wow" moments — things that I can do now that I couldn't do with hearing aids. If they had happened six months ago, I likely would have cried each time they happened. The happy tears are few these days and I think it's because hearing well has become the new "normal" for me. I'm not quite taking my good hearing for granted just yet but I can see it happening pretty soon. I still do smile when I realize how easy things are now but I have noticed that I'm actually beginning to pick out my "bad" moments more easily than my "wow" moments.

Hearing well at my office seems to be the easiest. I feel like a regular hearing co-worker now. I can hear and understand pretty much everything everybody else can. I walked down the hall and passed my boss's office. He was in a meeting. I heard him call my name and I turned around and went back. They all had big smiles on their faces because they wondered if I would come back. (Note to self: take off the CI while walking down the hall if you don't want to go to impromptu meetings.) I had my first web conference with my co-workers yesterday. We listened to a man on the speaker phone for an hour with no captions or anything. I could easily understand everything he and my co-workers said. I think back to all of the meetings I've been to in that conference room where I had to really read lips to understand my co-workers at the far end of the table and yet this meeting was so simple. Truly incredible.

I went on a chocolate tour in Beverly Hills on Saturday with my friend, Lori. It was an hour drive and I drove. I could easily understand Lori in the car without having to look at her. That's not a new "wow" but it still thrills me that I can do that, and that, too, is the new normal. We went to about six different shops on the tour, and each shop gave us a little spiel about what they sold there or a little history of their shop. I could easily understand what each person said, as well as the tour guide, even when I was preoccupied with scouring the huge selection of brownies.

We went geocaching after the tour. We went to a geocache that was outside the gates at Hugh Hefner's Playboy mansion. Several open air tour vans went by. I could easily hear the tour guides through the speakers but I wasn't always able to understand what they said. I think if I really tried to listen I might have done better. I did get a kick out of the tourist that turned around and took a picture of my Porsche. Several cars went through the gates, too. Each one had to talk to security on the intercom. I could hear both the people in the car and the security guy but I couldn't understand what they were saying. Lori could understand those conversations and the tour guides so she filled me in. Whenever situations like that happen when I still can't understand something, I simply ask myself if I could have done any better with my hearing aids and the answer is always "no." I doubt I would have been able to hear anybody on the intercom or the people in the cars.

I played MouseAdventure (a puzzle race in Disneyland) again on Sunday. The last time I played was when I only had one CI. I did do better this time. I actually heard my teammates call me back, and I was able to turn around and come back without them having to run after me. I understood all of them pretty easily. My friend, Jody, tends to not say very much but when she does it usually gets us a lot of points. I actually heard some of the things she said pretty easily and I think I might have missed them in the past as she speaks softly. I had difficulty understanding what was being said in the ballroom when they had the presentation. Could I have done better with my hearing aids? Definitely not, and, in fact, I understood much more than I did with my hearing aids.

The most important "wow" moment came after the race. I called my mom and gave her a recap of the chocolate tour and MouseAdventure. I normally use my older ear on the phone. Voices sound more normal in that ear so it is easier to understand what people are saying. It was about a 45 minute call and I did switch to my newer ear from time to time. It was when I listened to her munchkin voice in the newer ear and switched back to the older ear that I realized I was listening to my "old" mom. (Dang! *Now* I'm tearing up!) Her voice is the one voice I've been longing to hear the way I heard her with my hearing aids and that finally is happening now. It was especially evident using only the older ear. I had been told that people tend to hear voices more as they remember them as much as a year after getting a CI. It's been almost a year with my older ear so I guess they were right. Whenever I lose patience with my newer ear regarding voice quality, I listen to something with only my older ear and it gives me hope that the newer ear will get there, too, I just have to have more patience.

My brother, Steve, is going in for surgery tomorrow to get his second CI. He has made good progress with his first one but having two is so much better. I know he is going to love it. I can't wait for him to experience the new normal, as I am now.

October 6, 2013 Advanced Bionics Mentor Workshop

I just spent the past couple of days at Advanced Bionics for a Mentor Workshop. It was a very small group of only twenty-four mentors from around the country and Canada. I was honored to be asked to attend as they could only invite three mentors from our region and that includes all of Southern California, Arizona and New Mexico. I am the Chapter Leader of the brand new Orange County Chapter and that's why I was invited. I got to meet another Chapter Leader from Phoenix and another from the Bay area, as well. I got some great advice from them.

I am fortunate that Advanced Bionics is in Valencia, California. I was able to drive there while many people spent long hours on plane rides and in airports to attend. I got in about 8:45 pm on Thursday, and figured I would just go to my hotel room and spend the rest of the evening by myself. To my surprise, there was a representative from AB in the lobby lounge as well as several other mentors. I recognized one right away — Evelyn Gardner. She's a big name among the mentors and has provided me with a lot of help, so I was especially looking forward to meeting her in person. She was just as kind as I knew she would be. It turns out that a lot of the people had pretty late flights and they continued to trickle in through the evening. The first group went to bed and I went with the second group to the hotel next to ours for drinks. I had "met" several of them online through AB's forum, Hearing Journey, and on Facebook. We have also been in the Thursday night chats online but had never met in person before. It was really great finally getting to meet them in person. Needless to say, I didn't get to sleep until after midnight that night.

Friday was a full day with many different presentations. All of the speakers were really good and I was thrilled to meet even more people that I knew from online. I met some new people, too. At breakfast Friday morning, I met a mom of a child with a cochlear implant. Being the sap that I am, I started crying when it hit me just how fortunate her child is that he will not have to have the same experience growing up hard-of-hearing like Steve did. He is going to have a good shot at being a "normal" kid, and I am absolutely thrilled for him. It turns out there were about five parents of CI children there as mentors. What a great thing they are doing, making it easier for other parents to go through this journey. It was nice for them to talk to us, too, so that they could find out what their child is going through, since they obviously haven't gone through it themselves. After the day's presentations, we went back to the hotel for more drinks, a great dinner by AB, and more socializing late into the night. I sat with many different people so that I could meet as many as I could and hear their stories.

Saturday was a lot of fun. The President of the company came to talk to us. That's pretty impressive when you think about how big the company is and throw in the fact that it was a Saturday to boot. For him to take the time out of his schedule to talk to us shows just what a caring company AB is. He thanked us for what we do and answered all of our questions. He even posed for a picture with us. They had chocolate on the tables for us, but they really needed to have Kleenex. I cried as I thanked him for giving me my miracle and a couple of other people told him how their lives had changed. It was pretty emotional.

After we met him, we got together with our regional manager and the people from our own region and talked. Then we went on a tour of AB with our little group. I had asked, when I got there Thursday night, if they were giving the manufacturing tour and was pretty surprised that they didn't have time in the schedule. I told them they should do everything they could to add it since this was the first trip to AB for many of the mentors and it is really a great tour. I was very happy they were able to fit it in. I know it was a big highlight for many people. I was surprised to see so many people working on Saturday.

After that, we split up into groups of about eight for a few hours. We each filmed short videos that they will probably put on YouTube, or Facebook, or on their website. That was pretty fun. We also met with the web designer and gave some suggestions on how to improve the website, the forum, and the chat. I'm not sure how much they will actually be able to do but it was nice that they care, and that they want to continually improve things for us. Then we discussed our mentoring experiences with each other.

We had lunch and went back in with the whole group for the last presentation. Many people were flying home later that afternoon and evening. The session was interrupted when we were told that there was a fire on the freeway due to Santa Ana winds and that some people had to leave that very minute because the freeway was closed. Yikes! I had to take a detour driving home that added an hour to my commute but I went down a canyon that was absolutely gorgeous and had "Julie" roads with many twists and turns. I *loved* it. I only wish I had driven my Porsche. I may have to go on that road again in the spring when the hills are green. I was actually glad that the mentors had to take that detour because they at least got to see a pretty part of California instead of just the freeway and the hotel.

All in all it was an fantastic experience and I'm so glad I went.

October 23, 2013 # Las Vegas Trip

I went to Las Vegas with my cousin, Sue, a couple of weeks ago. We are avid geocachers and there was a big event being held there. Sue hadn't been to Las Vegas in thirty years so there was a lot for her to see and do. My new "wow" moments are few and far between now but that doesn't mean I don't appreciate what I'm hearing all the time.

It always amazes me that I can understand so well in the car now. Oh sure, I had to have Sue repeat herself occasionally, but it was not very often. I remember taking the same drive with my boyfriend just a year ago with my hearing aids and we didn't talk much the entire trip. It was too difficult to try to understand him and drive at the same time. I decided this would be a good chance to try out the new ZoomControl program on my Advanced Bionics Naida processor. I drove half the time on my regular program and then I drove the second half using the ZoomControl. It did sound a little bit different, but to be honest, I could hear so well without ZoomControl that it didn't make that much of a difference for me.

We went to a mini geocaching event on the first night at Fremont Street. It's a walking street downtown. There are lots of artists and street performers to watch as well as a great light show overhead that covers the entire street. The geocachers met in the middle to watch the light show together. I think I actually had an easier time understanding the people than my cousin did, due to my UltraZoom program. I am able to block out noise behind me and zoom in on the person in front of me. She wasn't so lucky.

We went to a couple of Cirque du Soleil shows – "LOVE" and "Zarkana." "LOVE" is all Beatles music. *Love* it, I did. It was a fantastic show. The sound system in there was incredible. There were even speakers in all of the seats and all of the seats were in the round. Surprisingly, the voices didn't bother me at all. I honestly don't remember if they sounded like the Beatles to me or not (it was the original recordings) but they must not have sounded bad because I thoroughly enjoyed it.

My brother, Steve, is getting his second implant turned on tomorrow. I have another friend that has only one implant that is considering whether or not to get a second one. She qualifies for it, but she's just not sure if she should get it. I took one of my CIs off to see how it would sound with only one ear. That didn't last long. I put it back on pretty quickly because it sounds so much better with two. Don't get me wrong, one CI sounds much better than two hearing aids. But if a person's hearing is bad enough that they qualify for two cochlear implants, it's definitely worth getting both of them. I can't wait for Steve to have his second ear.

I have to say that having lost my hearing and having gained it back has made me truly appreciate the fantastic sounds that I am hearing probably far more than regular hearing people do. I just couldn't get over how great that sound system was. One of the things that I have always loved about Cirque du Soleil shows is that they rarely talk. I have always been able to enjoy the performances as much as regular hearing people have. During the "LOVE" show, they did have some voiceovers where the Beatles spoke. I was very appreciative and amazed that I was able to understand what they said, even with their British accents. Both of them were great shows.

We went to Geocoinfest and had a great time there as well. They had a seminar where the geocaching reviewers answered peoples' questions. I had gone to GeoWoodstock with Sue when I had my hearing aids and they had the same seminar (obviously with different questions). When I was at GeoWoodstock, I couldn't understand hardly any of it. This time, however, I understood the majority of what the various reviewers said, and I was able to understand the questions that the various audience members asked. That was huge. The audience members didn't have microphones and I was not reading any lips. Many times the reviewers didn't use microphones either.

They also showed us about an hours' worth of geocaching films made around the world, maybe ten films in all. There weren't any captions but I think I understood the majority of the films. There were a couple of films that I had trouble with but I think that was more because I was fighting staying awake in the dark. Nobody has time to sleep in Vegas you know. We really enjoyed watching the films. Some of them were quite comical.

I had such a good time with my cousin. My ears have just made it that much easier and more relaxing. It's really nice not having to concentrate so hard trying to read lips.

October 26, 2013 Taste Buds and Renewed Hope for Music

One of the possible side effects of cochlear implant surgery is a loss or change of taste buds. This is supposed to be temporary but it can last a year or more. There are a lot of nerves in the area where they do the surgery and I guess it can take a while for them to heal. My first surgery was a year ago (still can't believe it's been that long already) and my second surgery was six months ago. I noticed an immediate change in my tongue after the first surgery. It was very smooth and slick. Water had a taste, not a bad taste, but a taste that wasn't there before. Some people have said they have a taste like metal and I suppose that would be as close of a description I could give you for water. You know how your mouth feels when you get up in the morning before you've brushed your teeth? Mine felt like that a lot. I would brush my teeth and then ten minutes later wonder if I had brushed my teeth yet. Bread, tortilla chips, and tortillas all tasted very dry like chalk or cotton or cardboard. This was amplified when I had my second surgery.

One of my favorite foods is chicken quesadillas. I remember having my first one at Chili's restaurant after my surgery. Steve likes them, too. We both got them. I remember telling him they were the worst I had ever had. They were very, very bland with very little taste. He said they were fantastic. Uh-oh. It was definitely me. I mistakenly ordered them again somewhere else and they were terrible there, too. I realized, then, that I was going to have to go without my beloved chicken quesadillas. Sigh. Fortunately, chocolate continued to taste great. Most other foods did, too.

When we were in Las Vegas a couple of weeks ago, we went to a Mexican restaurant and I ordered the chicken quesadillas (some habits are hard to break). To my surprise, they really tasted good. The other night I decided to try them at Chili's again. They were delicious. Yay! My taste buds have returned.

Music was something else that people told me could take a year or more before it started sounding good again. I have to admit, I gave up hope that voices would ever sound good in music again. My friend, David, who has had his CI for many years, told me not to give up, that it would come. That's easier said than done. Speaking voices sound human most of the time and I can tell people apart. They don't bother me at all. But singing voices tend to all sound the same. They aren't robotic or anything like that or monotone, but the characteristics that make voices different aren't there for me. Rod Stewart and Stevie Nicks, for example, have very unique voices. I was a huge fan of Carrie Underwood and Kelly Clarkson. With my CIs, however, they both sounded the same. In fact, *all* female singers sounded the same. It was as if only one female singer recorded every female song. Yesterday, a Stevie Nicks song came on the radio and I knew immediately it was her, not from the song but from her voice. Wow! I also heard the Doobie Brothers' "Black Water" which I haven't heard for years. I love that song. They sounded *great*. It was just like I remembered. I listened to some Adele songs last night and, except when she was in the higher ranges belting out her songs, she, too, had character. Yes! I have hope again. It's starting to come back with my taste buds.

One thing that I have enjoyed a lot with my CIs, is that I can understand more lyrics than I could before. When I was singing along to "Black Water" I realized I've been singing some of those lyrics wrong this whole time. The correct lyrics were quite clear on some parts. They make more sense, too. Ha! I have always loved music shows like *American Idol, The Voice*, and *X Factor* but I haven't had a lot of enthusiasm for them since I've gotten my CIs. In fact, I've got the new season of *The Voice* and *X Factor* on my DVR but haven't watched any of the episodes yet. I've considered just deleting them but I think I'll give them a try and see how they sound now.

I'm going to a chocolate festival today and, fortunately, I *know* everything there is going to taste fantastic. Yum! It's fabulous to have real, renewed hope for music, too!

November 6, 2013 One Year 'Ear'versary!

One year ago, today, I was activated on my first ear. Wow! Sure doesn't seem like it's been a whole year already. It's been quite an extraordinary year. Some benefits were expected but so many more weren't. Life is sure different for me now.

What I didn't count on was making so many friends. I have learned that people that were raised without hearing are "Deaf" and people like me, who have lost their hearing along the way, are "deaf." I have never belonged to the Deaf Community as I never considered myself Deaf or even deaf. I wouldn't even know how to join a Deaf Community. Steve was the only other person I knew with hearing loss as substantial as mine. Now I have many deaf and hard of hearing friends that have cochlear implants or are thinking about getting them. It's been really great to meet so many people that have been through my same experiences. Everybody "gets it" because we've all been there.

Being a mentor for Advanced Bionics has been a high point of my year. I'm doing something really worthwhile with my life and so many people appreciate the help that I have given them. It's been so little on my part, yet it seems to mean so much to so many. I get back just as much as I give. I've made some special friendships and it is so exciting to be there for each person's journey. I know what they have waiting for them, and it's so cool to be a part of it. I also think it's really neat that, being a Chapter Leader, I've been able to bring people together. I know a lot of friendships have been formed and that people look forward to seeing each other again at our socials. Quite frankly, I feel like a proud Mama.

I've always enjoyed public speaking and I always thought it would be really cool to be a professional motivational speaker. What a great job that would be. Well, I'm not a professional motivational speaker but I have been able to do more public speaking this past year. I know that my speeches have touched some people and I hope that my words can continue to help make a difference.

Of course, the obvious has happened. I can hear a whole lot better. I think I notice the change the most at work. I just can't tell you how great it is to be a "normal" co-worker again. It is so much easier now. I also love going to movies again. I never thought I would ever be able to understand them again in my life so that was a big one. Actually, I could go on and on about the things I love about it.

November 16, 2013 # HearAid Foundation Fundraiser

My surgeon, Dr. Jack Shohet, and my audiologist, Cheryl Tanita, are on the board of the HearAid Foundation. The foundation raises money to buy hearing aids for people that can't afford them. They had a fundraiser event last night. My friend, Jody, and I went. When we arrived, they had a lot of fun masks for us to choose from. I had to get the fanciest one that sparkled and had feathers, of course. Jody's mask was pretty, too, and matched her outfit.

It was held in the ballroom at the Islands Hotel in Newport Beach. There was a complimentary martini bar which made Jody quite happy. There were a lot of interesting silent auction items to bid on. Many items were autographed: a Fender guitar by The Rolling Stones, framed sheet music by Taylor Swift, a picture of Johnny Depp, a *Star Wars* poster, and even a record album signed by Michael Jackson. They had trips to New York, Cancun and even a trip to a Cubs game. There were a variety of other items to bid on, too. I bid on a massage but didn't win. It was fun to look at all of the items. They also had a photographer there taking our pictures.

After the cocktail hour, they opened the doors to the ballroom. We sat at a table with two other couples and had a delicious meal and nice conversation before the presentation. Our table was at the back of the room. In my hearing aid days that would have been cause for concern. We were too far from the stage for me to be able to read lips. In fact, I had been to Jody's daughter's wedding that was held in a hotel ballroom just a couple of months before my first ear was turned on. I vividly remember sitting there not hearing any of the funny speeches that were given. I know they were funny because I was the only one that wasn't laughing.

This time, not only was our seat too far from the podium, but there was also a large centerpiece on the table in front of us and it was directly in my line of sight of the presenters. To my delight, the emcee started talking and I understood everything she said. They showed a really nice video that had music playing and showed the various recipients of the hearing aids that the foundation was able to give out last year. I understood many of the words to the song. I did move to an empty seat on the other side of the table so that I could see the presenters but, again, it was too far to read their lips. There were about nine speeches in all and I understood all but two. Wow! It was so nice to be able to laugh with everyone else when one of the presenters told how his mother was not amused when he buried his first giant hearing aid from the 50's in the sandbox when he was a child. In my hearing aid days, that would have been a very long hour. But last night, I enjoyed it.

I have decided to do my part for the HearAid Foundation. Once people get a cochlear implant, they no longer wear their hearing aids. I am going to ask the people with CIs to bring their old hearing aids to the Bionic Ear Association gatherings. I would be thrilled to be able to present hearing aids to Dr. Shohet and Cheryl on a regular basis. I'm sure it would make the people that no longer need their hearing aids happy to be able to donate them to such a worthy cause, too. If you have hearing aids that are in good working order that you would like to donate or if you would like to make a monetary donation or learn more about the HearAid Foundation go to http://www.hearaidfoundation.org.

November 24, 2013 # Update on Steve

Yesterday was my mom's eighty-fifth birthday. My brothers, their wives, my dad and I took my mom out to Roger's Gardens to see all of their decorated Christmas trees, then to a yummy lunch at The Cheesecake Factory. I strolled through the gardens with Steve's wife, Shirley. She got pretty excited as she was telling me how much her life, as well as Steve's, has changed since he got his cochlear implants. He has had his first ear for eight months and his second for one month. She said he surprised her the other day when she sneezed in a different room than he was in. He said, "God bless you." she said, "Thank you" and he said, "You're welcome!" This is a little thing to those of you that can hear but it's a pretty big triumph for someone with a CI. I know how excited I get when I hear Bob opening the front door when I'm watching TV in the other room. I can hear his footsteps coming towards me and I call out, "Welcome home, Honey!" before he enters the room so I know how excited Steve must have been to hear that sneeze and to hear Shirley say, "thank you" — all from another room.

Their conversations are much easier now, too. Shirley used to have to speak very slowly and often had to repeat herself. She was often the interpreter for Steve when other people spoke to him, too. It wasn't unusual to find her finger spelling words to him that he didn't understand as well. Now, she said that she can talk just as fast as she talks to everyone else and rarely has to repeat herself. He's become a bit of a social butterfly, too. She's often surprised to find him going up to strangers and having conversations with them all on his own. That is *huge*. I think it's important to note that people with severe to profound hearing loss are often silent, and feel isolated, while others are conversing. I know I was. I often didn't hear the beginning of a conversation and didn't know what the topic was. I was also worried about answering a question wrong because I heard the question wrong to begin with. It's embarrassing! Sometimes it's easier to just be silent than to engage in conversation so that we don't make a fool of ourselves. For Steve to have the confidence to talk to people he doesn't know, without the need for Shirley to interpret, is astounding progress. He's also pre-diabetic and has begun a twelve week course on ways to prevent getting full blown diabetes. Shirley would have had to go with him in the past, but now Steve goes by himself. The teacher is Russian with a thick accent and he still understands her.

I sat next to him at The Cheesecake Factory. In the past, Steve was usually pretty quiet in restaurants. Not yesterday. He carried on quite a few conversations. It was pretty noisy in there, but Steve was telling my dad about the Advanced Bionics UltraZoom feature on his processor. It focuses the microphone on the people in front of him and lessens the sounds behind him. He could easily understand what was being said to him while it was actually harder for the rest of the family. He even told us a joke that one of my other brothers told him. It was actually a funny one for a change, too. Ha! He rarely understood my brother's jokes in the past and had to have them repeated and explained. Not anymore. He also told us how he heard the break bell at work for the first time recently. He has worked there for probably twenty years and had never heard it.

I love to hear him talk about how much he is enjoying music. Imagine living the last thirty-five years of your life without music. He remembers Olivia Newton John from his childhood. He listened to her, again, when he was first activated but she hasn't sounded good until now. He has the ComPilot, which is a Bluetooth that streams sound from devices like iPads, phones, etc. directly to the CI. He was listening to music with it but didn't like it at first. He said there were too many other sounds. I told him to have the audiologist set the ComPilot to 100% so that he wouldn't hear anything but what he was trying to listen to. He did, and now he loves it. He is especially partial to piano music now. I have been trying to get him to go to an instrumental concert with me but so far he won't. I'm going to keep trying, though, because I know how much he will enjoy it once he goes.

His life has changed so much in these past eight months and I know that it's going to continue to improve for at least another year if not more. I am beyond ecstatic for him. It is so incredible to be living in this day and age.

December 17, 2013 This and That

I realized I haven't written in almost a month. As my ears have become more and more "normal" there hasn't been too much "ear" news. I guess that's a good thing.

We did have our second Bionic Ear Association social this month. It was a whole lot easier this time than it was the first time. We moved it to Steve's clubhouse which is much larger and quieter. It rained pretty hard but that only kept one person away that was coming from the snow in Big Bear. I think that was understandable. It's so exciting to watch each person's progress. Some of the people that were there had just had surgery the first time we saw them, so it was neat to see how excited they were about what they could hear now.

Another woman had just had surgery. Still others were just starting the process or waiting for insurance approval. Waiting for the insurance approval is the hardest part of the entire process. Well, the most agonizing anyway! I love to see the friendships form and I love to see Steve being so social. He was talking and helping so many people.

I went to Disneyland today with a truly great friend, Jody. A great friend will humor you when you want to do a hearing experiment and ride the same ride two times in a row even though there's a long line. One item that is still left unchecked on my hearing wish list is to be able to hear the characters' voices on the different rides. We went on the Pirates of the Caribbean ride. Unfortunately, the couple to my right and the person behind me talked the majority of the time on our first time through. I had my processor on my "widest" program — the one that allows the widest range of sound to come through. Unfortunately, it was too loud. It picked up all of the sounds, which was too much for me. Part of it was pretty cool because at the very beginning of the ride you can hear birds, frogs, bugs and a banjo. I've heard the frogs before, but I don't remember hearing some of the high-pitched birds. I also noticed that the skull at the beginning of the ride changed what he said. I remember that he told us to keep our hands and arms inside the boat the last time but now he mentioned something about Davey's Locker (I think). I also noticed that they used to play the pirate song more and now they say "deeeaaaad men tell tallll tales" (I think) an awful lot. Other than that I only heard Johnny Depp say "magnificent" at the very end of the ride.

I asked Jody if she'd mind riding again so that I could switch my processor to a program that allowed less sound in. Being the good friend that she is, she agreed. Fortunately, we were in the last seat and nobody talked this time. Unfortunately, that seat is very wet. I realized early on I still wasn't going to understand the words so I did a different experiment instead. I closed my eyes through most of the ride and decided to see if I could hear where the voices and sounds were coming from. Sure enough, sometimes they were on my right, sometimes on the left and sometimes they were straight ahead or overhead. Having two ears allows me to be able to do this. I have to say, it's pretty cool.

We went on a couple more attractions. Tarzan's tree house has changed it seems. We also went on the single rider line on Indiana Jones and got right on. It was a great way to avoid a *long* line. I had two free tickets to see the movie *Frozen* so we went to see that, too, in Downtown Disney. I got the closed caption device but it didn't work. It didn't matter. I didn't need it. That was especially good because it was an animated movie with songs, no less. I'm finding that I'm using closed captioning less and less. I watched the entire *Survivor* finale and reunion show at a friend's house the other night and didn't need the captioning at all. I understood probably 98% of the shows. Man, that's a great feeling!

I crossed off one more item from my wish list this month. I finally heard my cat purr.

December 25, 2013 # Being Normal

Life with a cochlear implant still presents its challenges. There are definitely times when I know that I am still deaf. I went to see *The Nutcracker* last week with some old friends. Dinner was a little hard with music playing in the background, tile floors, and six of us around the table. I was deaf again in the lobby of the theater with people chattering all around. Although those situations were no worse than it was when I wore hearing aids, I knew I wasn't normal like the rest of them were. I did enjoy the performance. The music was fantastic and I loved seeing my friend's daughter, Bella, dance in the show. Of course, I wouldn't have traded seeing my friends again for anything. That part was priceless. I think what hearing people don't realize is how much energy and stress is involved in lipreading and filling in the blanks of words that are missed. It can be frustrating and tiring.

I also got to go on two hikes this week, each with a different friend— Marsha and Jeremy. On each of those hikes I was *completely* normal. I had no hearing handicap whatsoever. I used to dread parts of the trail where we had to go single file. It's impossible to read lips when someone is in front of you or behind you. Not this time. It didn't matter where we were in relation to each other. I didn't have to read lips at all. I was free to enjoy the beautiful views all around me while still participating in the conversations. I heard the birds all around. At one point I did have to ask Jeremy what I was hearing. It was a constant pounding sound and I wasn't sure if it was a woodpecker or not. He pointed out some kids playing in a tree a couple hundred feet away. Aha! Jeremy and I went to a restaurant afterwards and, because we got there around 3:00 pm, there was nobody else around. Again it was completely normal. No lipreading was required, and I understood every word.

Marsha and I went to a geocaching event after our hike. It was in a park in the evening. In the past I would have been a bit anxious. Once the lights go dim it's extremely difficult for a person with hearing aids to hear. People with hearing aids actually hear more with their eyes than their ears. When it gets hard to see, lipreading becomes very difficult. It didn't matter there. I was hearing with my ears, no longer with my eyes. I was able to participate in the conversations even though it was dark. Even though there were a lot of people there, it wasn't noisy. Once again, I was normal.

An old co-worker of mine is on Facebook. She reminded me how much I struggled back in those days. I was in my twenties then. I'm forty-eight now. That was in the early days of my hearing loss. I then thought about college and how difficult that was. They didn't have cochlear implants back then. I think about all of the young people that are getting cochlear implants now and how they, too, are going to live so much of their lives feeling normal and I am filled with overwhelming emotion of joy and gratitude for how much easier their life is going to be than it was for me. A senior friend of mine who wears hearing aids told me she was too old to get a cochlear implant. Nonsense! That woman has more spunk and life in her than many people half her age. Even if she only has five years left to live (and I'm sure she has many more than that) what better way to live them than to be able to hear again for the rest of her life? What a gift that would be.

2013 has been a real blessing for me. I'm looking forward to what the new year has to bring.

January 19, 2014 Stampin' Up! Leadership Conference

I went to Houston a couple of weeks ago for the Stampin' Up! Leadership Conference with my friend, Glad. It was very similar to my convention experience that I wrote about on July 29, 2013. This time, though, I decided to sit in the regular seats and not in the "special needs" section. Normally, the special needs section is in front of the teleprompter and I always had that as a backup to read if I couldn't understand a presenter. This time, the seats were behind the teleprompter so that wouldn't have worked even if I needed it. I didn't have the anxiety I had at convention, because I knew I could understand the presenters the last time. Sure enough, I understood them all this time, too. The difference, though, was that they had a keynote speaker this time. I have seen many keynote speakers and have sat in the audience many times when everyone around me laughed and laughed and I just sat there. I rarely understood what they were saying and they never use a teleprompter. I was a bit excited to see if I could finally laugh along with everyone else. Yes! I did. It was fantastic to be able to hear their jokes from beginning to end and actually do a real laugh with the crowd. I couldn't believe it. I thought I was through crying over my "wow" moments but evidently I'm not. People must have thought there was something wrong with me crying while everyone else was laughing. I'm such a sap.

Another surprising realization occurred during our lunches. We sit at large round tables with about six people at each table. With hearing aids, I could pretty much only understand the people sitting right next to me. I could read lips, of course, and try to get the rest but it was always hard. This time, with my UltraZoom program, I was able to understand and converse with everyone at the table with no anxiety.

I did a little sightseeing on my own the day before the conference. I took a lot of buses and would tell the bus drivers where I wanted to get off. It was nice to be able to hear them tell me when to get off the bus. I saw lots of interesting things: the Holocaust Museum, a house made entirely of beer cans, beautiful gardens, neat sculptures, and busts of all of the presidents that stood about eight feet tall. You can see them behind The Beatles statues which were thirty feet tall. Fun!

When I went back to work last week, the auditors from Taiwan were there. They are very soft-spoken, have accents, and their English is not always the best. Usually, I would have to ask them to repeat themselves many times. This time, I could actually hear them and even understood what they were saying, but I still had to ask them to repeat themselves to try to understand their meaning in what they were trying to say. But it was nice being able to actually have the volume to really hear them the first time. I took them to the beach one evening and I was able to understand them speaking to me while I was driving. I wouldn't have been able to do that before. At least that was a bit easier, too.

February 10, 2014 Great End to a Very Stressful Week!

Last Monday I had to do probably one of the hardest things I've ever had to do in my life. We had to put my dad, who has Alzheimer's and can no longer walk, into a home. We took him to the hospital to have his legs checked out and afterwards the hospital didn't recommend that he go back home. I was on the phone so much on Monday that my battery was almost dead by the time I got home late that night. I am extremely grateful for my CI, as I was able to understand the majority of the phone conversations and I was able to get everything taken care of that I needed to do, including contacting the 911 operator to get an ambulance for Dad.

Needless to say, the earlier part of the week was pretty tough on our family. As the week went on, it got better. The place the hospital recommended is really a great place and Dad seems to be adjusting quite well, all things considered. Of course, he would much rather be home, but he is enjoying the activities that they have and he's getting lots of visits from the family. They give him a lot of desserts, too.

I had made plans to go to the Hollywood Museum with my friend, Lori, on Saturday. By that time, I was ready for some fun so we went. It was a pretty neat museum with lots of movie and TV memorabilia. They had items from when I was a kid all the way through current shows that are on TV now.

We finished pretty fast, though, and wondered what to do next. Just then a guy came and gave us half off of a Hollywood sightseeing tour. Since we didn't have anything else to do and since we were being tourists anyway, we decided, "Why not?" We went on a two hour tour through Hollywood and Beverly Hills. The driver was also the tour guide, which means we could not see him while he spoke. In the olden days, that would have meant a two hour tour just enjoying the views but not having any clue whose homes we were seeing. Not this time. I understood probably 95% of what he said *and* he even had an accent. It was *great*.

I decided that my mom really needed a break, too. We treated ourselves to the Glen Ivy Spa on Sunday. The weather wasn't very good when we got there, but by the time we had a relaxing massage, and then a fantastic facial after that, the clouds cleared. We ate lunch, changed into our bathing suits and hit the outdoor Jacuzzi. I brought along my Neptune processor which is completely waterproof. Whenever we've gone to Glen Ivy in the past, I was always deaf for the majority of the day. If my hair was wet, I couldn't wear my hearing aids. Not this time. I was able to enjoy our time together in the Jacuzzi without having to read Mom's lips and I didn't have to worry about the water or having wet hair. After that, I went to the lounge pool and floated around there while listening to all of the sounds going on around me. It was quite a different experience.

It was so nice to be able to hearing everything over the weekend after having such a stressful week. I'm also grateful I was able to make all of the arrangements that I needed to make on the phone on Monday, too.

February 12, 2014   Human Voices and Song Lyrics

One of the biggest fears that people have about getting a cochlear implant is that they will not hear voices the way they hear them with their hearing aids. I certainly had that fear as well. If you remember, I heard voices as if everyone was on helium when I was first activated. My dad sounded like a five-year-old girl back then. Some people hear beeps for speech, some hear robotic voices, etc. With time and practice, the voices slowly change.

A friend of mine that has a CI asked if the voices were ever going to sound "normal". I hadn't really thought about it in a while so I paid particular attention to the sound of the voices as I was watching TV. It actually caught me off guard that every character sounded exactly as I remembered them. I knew voices were better. I have had "wow" moments along the way when I longed to hear particular peoples' voices the way I remembered them and finally did, but it kind of snuck up on me that everybody sounds normal now.

Voices in music still aren't the way I remember them but it's coming along. I had a different "wow" moment with music today. I haven't used my Compilot for a few months. I used it at work today to listen to Pandora music on my phone for a few hours. I could not believe just how many lyrics I understood. I have been hearing words and phrases here and there when I listen to music in the car but I actually understood probably 75% of an Adele song and quite a bit of a lot of others. These are songs that I don't know the words to, by the way. On songs that I do know the words to, the lyrics are very clear.

It just keeps getting better and better, and more and more "normal" all the time!

March 4, 2014 My Dad

It's with a heavy heart that I tell you that my dad has pneumonia and only days left to live. My CIs have come through for me yet again, but this time during a very difficult time in my life. Dad went into the ICU on Friday. My brothers and I decided to take shifts staying with him in the hospital. I volunteered to stay with him at 1:00 am. That first night I stayed awake the whole time, as he kept waking up and needed me often. The second night, I came at 1:00 am again. I hadn't gotten much sleep and was pretty exhausted when I got there. My brother that I relieved said that Dad was sleeping soundly. I decided to take advantage of the padded bench in his room and lay down. I kept my CI on and closed my eyes. I was able to hear Dad breathing. I could also hear whenever anyone came into the room. I was easily able to open my eyes to check on Dad and to help the hospital staff deal with him.

That was a real blessing to me. I never would have been able to do that when I wore hearing aids. I would have had to stay awake and alert the whole time which, as tired as I was, would have been impossible to do.

The next day there was pretty much a party in his room. There were fourteen loved ones all crammed in his room. Unfortunately, I had to take a call from one of the hospital administrators on the phone in Dad's room. That would have been impossible with my hearing aids. With my CI, I answered the phone with confidence. I took the headpiece of one of my processors off my head so that I would be completely deaf in that ear and listened to the phone with my other ear. To my delight and surprise, I was able to handle the entire conversation without having to shush anybody. There were multiple conversations going on all around me and I was able to take care of what needed to be done very easily. If I had been wearing my hearing aids, I probably wouldn't have been able to hear on the phone at all — even in a quiet room. If I could hear, I definitely would have needed silence around me, and I likely would have had to have the person repeat themselves multiple times.

Dad is home from the hospital now and I have been fortunate to spend a lot of time with him. There are times that he barely whispers but I am able to hear him. Time is drawing to an end but I will always be able to remember "I love you more" whispered from my dad thanks to my CI.

April 3, 2014 Beeps for Speech and Reverberation

I thought I'd give a little hope to those of you that are in the earlier stages of having a cochlear implant who might be hearing beeps for speech or reverberation. I was one of the lucky "rock stars" that only heard beeps for speech for just a few seconds during my activation. Much to my surprise, I heard those same beeps for speech many months later. It was when I was listening to something and the volume was so low that I could just barely hear any sound and I was straining to hear. This makes a lot of sense when you think about it. If you take a look at my audiology exam from before I had my CI, you'll see my hearing was way at the bottom of the scale.

To help you understand how serious that loss is, even with hearing aids, I had to have the volume all the way up on the TV. Even then I couldn't understand it. I had to wear headphones and have captions on. In the first few weeks (or even longer) of having a CI, the brain begins to adapt and quickly craves more, and more, and more volume until it is hearing what a normal person hears.

There is a period where the CI processor is straining to hear, yet it is very loud for the person wearing the CI for the first time. If you set the volume on the CI at the normal person's range on day one, it would be like blowing your eardrum out. It would be way too much for the brain to handle. You have to grow into it. That's why, I believe, some people hear beeps instead of speech in the early days of wearing their CI. The volume is too low for the CI to properly process speech, yet very loud for the new CI user. It goes away as the brain adapts to the higher volume.

As for the reverberation, I never had that problem, yet I have heard about it from many new CI users. I finally heard it when I was watching the movie *Saving Mr. Banks*. I could understand the majority of the movie until the very end. In the last scene, they show a tape recorder and it is playing the original tapes. It was loud enough, but I could not make out what was being said. That entire scene was with reverberation. That, too, made a whole lot of sense to me. It is normal for new CI users not to understand speech in the beginning. My theory is that when speech becomes clear, the reverberation goes away. I decided to test this theory on my friend, who regularly was complaining of reverberation. There is a great rehab exercise that I always recommend to new CI users. When you read along while listening to audiobooks, speech is usually clear. If you just listen without reading along, that same speech is not able to be made out. I asked my friend, who had the horrible reverberation, if she still had it when she read along with her audiobooks and the answer was no. When speech was clear there was no reverberation.

If ever there was a reason to work diligently on rehabbing a new CI ear, that was it. If you are having these problems, know that there is hope that they will go away as the brain adapts and speech becomes more understandable. You can help that along by doing rehab exercises. Reading along while listening to audiobooks for thirty minutes a day really helps. I also have a daily Facebook rehab group where I post four exercises a day: phone, audio, Angel Sound program (word exercises) and an "other" exercise which consists of various apps, websites, music exercises, etc. Anyone with a CI is welcome to join the group. Do a search for Cochlear Implant Daily Rehab and you will find it.

Note that there is no proof to my theories (that I am aware of anyway) and, although I believe them to be true, this is just my opinion.

April 8, 2014 I'm Still deaf

I went out to dinner and then to The Improv (comedy club) the other night. The Improv has always been a tough one for me. Nothing's worse than understanding the first part of a joke and missing the punchline, especially when you can hear the laughter all around and you know you missed a good joke. I guess I'm a glutton for punishment because I still like to go in hopes that, just maybe, I'll be able to understand the jokes from start to finish. At least with my cochlear implants I had hope. Unfortunately, that hope was not to be turned into reality . . . this time! There were three comedians that night. It was almost like the story of the three bears. The first comedian was a woman and her voice was a little too high. I got some of her jokes. I know she has size double A boobs. The second comedian was a man whose voice was a little too deep. I didn't get much of anything he said but he must have been very funny because the place was laughing like crazy. The headliner comedian was just right. I understood a lot of what he said but not everything. You would think that understanding 50% wouldn't be so bad, right? Well, it would be okay if I understood 100% of one joke, 0% of the next one, etc., but not when you hear only half of each joke. Fortunately, I did get most of the last comedian's jokes from start to finish or at least enough that I could fill in the blanks.

Oh well. What it did do was make me realize that, yep, I'm still deaf. It also reminded me of where I've been. That's not such a bad thing. As a mentor, and Chapter Leader of the Bionic Ear Association it's a good thing to remember what that's like. It's important not to forget. It's easy to take my bionic ears for granted these days.

It also helped me to appreciate just how far I've come. The next day I went to Borrego Springs for the weekend. It's about a three hour drive to get there. I drove and had three passengers with me. I easily looked straight ahead and had a long conversation with my mom in the seat next to me. I could also easily understand the conversation my boyfriend was having with my brother in the back seat. When I go to lunch with my brothers and co-worker twice a week, I sit in the back seat. I can now easily understand what the conversation is in the front seat. I couldn't do that a year ago.

I like to go hiking with a group of friends. I can't help but smile and be amazed each and every time I go out with them because I can understand the conversations going on around me now. I appreciate it so much every single time we go. It's so nice to be able to go on a narrow trail, single file, and still be able to understand what's being said. I used to only be able to understand the person next to me and had to read their lips. I don't have to do that any more and haven't for a while now. If there were three of us, forget it. I had a really hard time getting those conversations.

So yes, I'm still deaf. Some places are just like old times. But that's okay because boy, have I come a long way. And, yes, I still have hope that some day I'm going to be able to go to The Improv and laugh with everybody else.

May 17, 2014 Find the Positives

I remember one time when I took my young nephew, Joel, to Legoland. It was just the two of us and we were stuck in a very long line. We quickly got very bored and weren't having a very good time. I decided I didn't want to be bored and looked around for something positive about the situation. There were a lot of different people in that line. I started making up little back stories on each person in the line. One man was actually a Russian spy. A mother of three was actually a jewel thief. An old woman with a cane wasn't really an old woman. That was just her disguise. She was really a federal agent after the spy and the jewel thief. That cane wasn't really a cane either. It could shoot bullets. I also made a rule that each time something happened, and I can't remember what, we had to spin around in a circle. Being in that line might have been the most fun we had that day.

Joel is a teenager now and he's enjoyed writing stories for a while. He even told me he put me as a character in one of them but he hasn't let me read it. Hmmm, do you think he killed me off? I know this is probably going to be hard for you to believe, but yes, I *am* the crazy aunt in the family.

As a mentor, I have met a lot of really great people and I have been along their journey the whole way. I vividly recall one person, in particular, who was having a really difficult time with their rehab. According to them, they just were not doing well at all. They did everything I recommended that they do but they just weren't getting better. I finally asked what scores they were getting and which level they were on in the Angel Sound program they were working on. They were getting 85% on level four which is one of the hardest levels you could be on. They were scoring higher than I was. Needless to say, I was shocked. This person was being way too hard on themselves. Fortunately, I had the person keep a hearing journal all along the way where they had to write down all of the things they could hear that they couldn't hear before as well as the things they were having difficulties with. I had them read that journal and they admitted that there were many things they could do now that they had difficulties with in the beginning. They realized that they actually *had* come a long way from where they started.

Sometimes you have to stop and ask yourself a few questions. Am I doing everything I should be doing? Am I putting in the time to do the rehab? Am I wearing my CI without the hearing aid sometimes? If you are, then your negative emotion isn't helping you. It's time to change that emotion and think about your progress. Think about all of those baby steps along the way because they matter! Think about where you started out. How far would you have been on that program with your hearing aids? You probably couldn't even hear it. Think about all of the sounds you've heard: leaves crunching, birds singing, elevator bells dinging, doors closing in the other room. Write that list and read that journal. Instead of thinking "I *only* got 85%." say "Wow! I got 85%! I only got 4% with my hearing aids!" If you truly are doing what you should be doing, then beating yourself up isn't going to do any good. Our CIs *are* miracles but it's not a change that is immediate. It takes time, practice, patience and persistence. On the other hand, if you've given up on therapy and you aren't improving, then beating yourself up may give you the motivation to think about where you could be and it might bring about the change you need.

I was recently tested and got 94% in speech recognition. Needless to say, I was thrilled. But that didn't happen overnight. I worked very hard every day for a long time to get there. The rewards were well worth the time and effort.

It's important to learn to recognize when you are having emotions that aren't helping you. You *can* turn those emotions around. Simply ask yourself: Do I like feeling this way? Is feeling this way going to bring about positive change? If the answer to those two questions are no, then work on changing your attitude. Try to find something positive in the situation that you are in. Don't be too hard on yourself. You'll lead a much happier life, and your family and your co-workers will be happier, too.

May 17, 2014 Being Bilateral

I'd like to share how my experience with being bilateral (having two CIs) has been. Originally, I had only planned on having one ear done. I planned to save my good ear until better technology came along. I had heard about stem cell research and wanted to hold out for that. My surgeon had suggested that I get my second ear done six months after the first. I qualified for both. He told me that any new way of hearing was ten years away and more likely twenty years by the time it became widespread use. He also told me that the longer I waited the worse my auditory nerve was going to be, which meant that it would be harder for me to adapt to a CI or another way of hearing. Of course, that also meant my hearing would also deteriorate over time as well. Well, I was a hearing aid user then. I didn't have my first CI yet, and we all know that we can hear "just fine" with our hearing aids. I'm sure you can relate. So, I decided not to take his advice. I talked to my audiologist and she told me that they would be testing my hearing annually and that if she noticed any change that she would let me know and I could do it then. That sounded good to me.

Then I got my CI and I wore it by itself, without the hearing aid. I was amazed at how much better it was than my hearing aid. I then read Arlene Romoff's book, *Listening Closely: A Journal to Bilateral Hearing* about her decision to go bilateral and I knew that I had to do it *now*. Although my CI was fantastic, there were still a few drawbacks to only using one ear and she could do those things that I still couldn't. She also talked about her internal implant failing. She only had one CI at the time, which meant that she was completely deaf in her implanted ear until she could get the insurance approval, had the surgery, and waited for activation. When you come from hearing aids to getting a CI, it's not so bad because your hearing aids are pretty useless anyway and you have been reading lips for a long time. But when you come from good hearing with a CI to going deaf, it's deafening for lack of a better word. With a second CI, you would never be completely deaf again. You would always have a backup ear that worked well.

I went ahead with the surgery and got my second implant six months later as my surgeon had recommended. I'll never forget driving to work in my Porsche right after I got the second ear. I put on my favorite Styx CD and tears poured down my face for a solid half hour on that drive. I had forgotten just how awesome listening to music in stereo sounded! There are speakers in the front and the rear and certain songs had different instruments coming out of different speakers. Sometimes the sound traveled around from speaker to speaker. It was truly fantastic. You definitely don't get that with just one CI.

Another fantastic feature was that I no longer had to position myself so that people were on my CI side. I didn't have to sit in optimal listening position at dinner. I could sit anywhere and people could talk to me from both sides. It didn't matter if I was the driver or the passenger. I was not going to be at a disadvantage in either position.

I also hated changing my Neptune batteries because when they died, I was deaf. The same was true with changing programs. It wasn't a long time, but if I was listening to someone and I wanted to change programs I either had to ask them to wait a minute or read lips until the next program turned on. I have disabled the Quick Sync feature on my Naidas so that I can change programs on one ear and still hear fine out of the other ear. I no longer have to worry about timing the program change just right or interrupt conversations to change programs or batteries.

My comprehension is better with two ears as well. The sound is much fuller with two. The strange thing is that if I wear each one by themselves, voices are still a bit high pitched. But when I wear them together, voices sound much more normal. I don't know why that is, but it is.

I was also concerned about insurance. I had really good insurance through work at the time. I knew that with the changes in healthcare that my employer might have to scale back on our plan and who knows what insurance will be like ten years from now. I knew that I qualified now and was approved for the second ear, and decided I'd better not take that for granted.

I'm not sure if you are familiar with Rush Limbaugh. He is a famous talk radio personality. He got his first CI thirteen years ago. He, too, decided he would wait for better technology before getting his second ear done. They told him it would be ten years away. Well, it's been thirteen years and they are still telling him it will be ten years away. He realized that he wasted thirteen years of good hearing and he was not going to wait any more. He just had his second CI surgery.

Going bilateral was a great decision!

May 22, 2014 Visit to the Dentist and Afternoon Tea

Here's a very simple way to test your hearing — go to the dentist and get your teeth cleaned. If you can understand everything they say to you, then you probably have perfect hearing. When I had my hearing aids, I couldn't understand anything they told me. They would have to lower their mask to talk to me. There was no hope if they were behind me.

I've had my first cochlear implant for eighteen months now and the second one for a year. In fact, my one year anniversary of my activation was a week ago. The "wow" moments aren't coming anymore. My hearing is probably about as good as it's going to get at this point. So I was caught a bit off guard when I got all emotional at the dentist this morning. I was sitting in the chair facing the window. Music was playing pretty loud. The next thing I knew, the dental assistant is asking a bunch of questions from behind me. I doubt I would have even known she was in the room before. I answered all of her questions very easily. She told me all kinds of things about my teeth from behind her mask while she was doing the cleaning. I understood every word. This isn't the first time I've been to the dentist when I've heard every word, but it still never ceases to amaze me that *I'm getting every word!* Each time she says something to me, I realize anew, I'm hearing every word until my eyes are swelling up with tears and, sure enough, they start to flow. The poor girl thinks she's hurting me so she stops and asks me if I'm okay. Well, then that really gets me crying as I explain to her that they are happy tears. This is a new assistant who hasn't met me before. She thought it was pretty cool, too.

Why does this get to me when regular conversations don't? I'm hearing regular conversations just as well as I heard her but there are visual cues. I can see mouths move and I can read expressions. These visual cues have helped people with various stages of hearing loss "hear" for years. Most people with hearing loss use their eyes to hear and not their ears. So when you take away all of those cues with a mask, or by standing behind a person while talking, you truly realize that you are definitely hearing with your ears and not your eyes anymore. I've known I've been doing it for a while now, but the dentist is always the true test and it still shocks me that I can pass that test with flying colors.

I also smiled to myself yesterday as I realized *I'm getting every word!* in a very difficult listening environment. I went to tea with four of my friends. This particular tea house was especially noisy as there was a screaming baby there. I had already turned my UltraZoom program on that allowed me to focus on sound coming from in front of me and lowered the background sounds. I also lowered the volume one beep. I had very little problem understanding any of the conversations. My friends, however, kept commenting on how loud it was in there and finally, the manager asked them to remove the baby so that the rest of the place could enjoy their afternoon tea.

May 28, 2014 Breast Cancer Scare

This chapter is just a tiny portion about my cochlear implants but it's an important enough topic that I thought it deserved a chapter anyway. I am going to get the "girls" put through the torture chamber this morning. This is also known as getting a mammogram. I'm forty-nine years old and I've been getting them since I was about forty. I think most women start when they are fifty. I have a cousin on my dad's side that had breast cancer when she was young and my dad's mother also had cancer so I asked to start having them early. They didn't want to at first but I persisted. I'm sure glad I did!

The first few that I had were normal. But then one time I got the dreaded call back that they might have seen something and that I needed to go to the hospital to get another one since they have the best equipment there. But they were sure that it was "nothing" and not to worry about it. So I went. They had me wait after the test was done so that the doctor could take a look at it. Sure enough, they still saw "something" and wanted me to have an ultrasound "just to be safe" and that "for most people it's nothing so you really don't have anything to worry about." Yeah, okay. Now ultrasound technicians won't tell you anything because that's the doctor's job. But I could see the look in her eyes and it wasn't "nothing to worry about."

Yep, I needed to take the next step right away. I had to have a biopsy done. "But don't worry. Very few people have anything wrong and it's just a precaution. There's nothing for you to worry about. How soon can you have it done?" I seemed to be the "winner" in the "very few people" so far so, needless to say, I really didn't like hearing that and I *was* definitely worried. Sure enough, I had reason to be. The biopsy didn't come back as full on cancer but it wasn't "nothing" either. I had suspicious cells that would have to be removed surgically.

I'm normally a very positive person, and I try not to jump to conclusions, especially about something as important as the big "C": Cancer. That was my first surgery. It was only outpatient surgery and not a very big deal. I've had surgery to remove part of my colon, and two cochlear implant surgeries since then, but having those cells removed was the hardest surgery I've ever had. The mental anguish is excruciating. It seemed like *forever* until I got the results. So many awful things went through my mind even though I would tell myself not to go there because it might be taken care of. It turned out to be good news. I only had precancerous cells but if I had left them undetected, they may have turned into full blown breast cancer. It turns out that mammogram may have saved my life or, at the very least, my breast.

I had to have an MRI every six months for a couple of years after that. I know a lot of people get freaked out by them, but having a profound hearing loss worked out in my favor. They told me I had to wear ear plugs, but believe me, I didn't hear anything during the twenty minutes I had to lay there. It was so peaceful, in fact, that I was worried I would fall asleep and jerk and have to start over. You have to lay extremely still in there. I would sing to myself in my mind to stay awake. Once I put my hearing aids back on and was back in the dressing room I could hear just how loud those machines were. Yikes!

I was very grateful when the day came that they told me I could go back to having annual mammograms. I am even more grateful every time that they tell me it's fine and to come back next year.

When it came time for me to consider getting my first cochlear implant, one of the first things that came to mind was my breast history and the fact that you can't have an MRI with a cochlear implant. Well, you can, but they have to remove the magnet inside your head first. It's not as simple as just taking the processor off. I called my breast surgeon and asked her opinion. She told me that if it should come back that there were other ways that they could test me. I could still have CT scans and she was sure that they could make it work. She said the quality of my life would be greatly enhanced by the CI and that was more important than the ability to have an MRI. She encouraged me to move forward with it. I was relieved to have my breast surgeon's blessing.

I found out later that yet another one of my cousins on my dad's side also had breast cancer. These were young women. My heart goes out to both of them and to all women that have or have had breast cancer. It's the scariest thing I've ever dealt with in my life and I've dealt with some scary stuff. Ladies, I *strongly* encourage you to get on the phone *today* and make an appointment for a mammogram if you haven't had one or if you are overdue for getting one. They *can* save your life!

Note: Now you *can* get MRIs with some cochlear implants.

June 15, 2014 Prized Possession for You and Your Kids

This chapter is only about 1% related to my hearing. However, it's something that I feel strongly about so I thought I would share, especially because it is Father's Day. My father passed away in March. He had Alzheimer's. About seven years ago I had one of the best ideas I've ever had in my life. I'm about to pass that idea on to you in hopes that you will use it.

My family has always taken home movies but they are usually of somebody opening a Christmas gift or waving hello to the camera — nothing of any real substance. There are often times when I wish I could talk to my grandparents. They all died when I was fourteen or younger so I didn't much think about these kinds of things at that age. But as an adult, I realize that they lived through some interesting times and there are so many things I wish I could have asked them. I realized that some day my two nephews might also have those questions and wished they had asked my parents. Shoot, *I* might wish I had asked my parents certain things some day.

I also really wanted to capture my "real" parents and not my "video" parents. I wanted to capture the way they really talk, their mannerisms, the way they interacted with each other, etc. I wanted to have their "real" voices that I could listen to after they were gone. I came up with the idea to have a DVD series of interviews. Steve agreed to be the camera man and I set about making up a great deal of interview questions. I gave my parents a copy of the questions ahead of time so that they could think about their answers. I also asked them to dig up any pictures or mementos they had that related to the questions. It took several weekends and we wound up with four separate DVDs: one on my mom's early years; one on my dad's early years; one on their teenage years together (they met as teenagers); and one on inventions that they lived through.

I asked questions about everything I could think of starting back as far as they could remember like who their parents and grandparents were and what they did for a living as well as who their own siblings were. I asked questions about what their favorite things to do were, what their hobbies were, where they went to school plus their favorite and least favorite subjects, what kind of student they were, what they did after school, what their first job was and how they got it, how they met, how they learned to drive, and how they got their first car, etc. Since they were teenagers during World War II I asked questions about how the war affected them. Dad was drafted so he talked at length about what he did in the Army and about the letters he and Mom wrote to each other — in Morse Code no less. They lived through lots of inventions: the change from "ice boxes" to refrigerators, changes in telephones, the first TV, and more. I asked them about all of those things.

Each answer was always much more detailed than I had originally imagined and often veered off track, but that's how Dad told his stories anyway, so that was certainly him. I captured his "Hold on! Hold on! Hold on!" gestures as he stopped Mom when she was talking about "making out" with him, as he wanted us to know that "making out" in those days did *not* mean they had sex. It was just "necking". He got emotional talking about how much the daily letters he received from my mom meant to him while he was in the service, and about how he thought for sure she was going to leave him when she saw that he had lost a lot of hair while he was away. It was beautiful to see the love in their eyes as they talked about their early dates.

The intent of the DVDs, when I came up with the idea, was that they were mainly for me to watch after they were gone. I had no idea that they would actually be beneficial for Dad, too. As I said before, Dad had Alzheimer's. He forgot quite a lot about his life. One day I decided to invite him over to watch the DVD of his early years. He was fascinated. He forgot so many of those things that just five years earlier he could recall so vividly. He was amazed that the drawings he was holding up on the DVD were drawings he drew himself. I was really glad that we were able to give some of those memories back to him — in his own words no less. I'm sure he forgot them quickly afterwards but, for the moments that he watched the DVD, they were real.

Today is Father's Day. Dad had Alzheimer's for so long and had changed so much that "Old Dad" actually passed away a long time ago and "New Dad" took his place. I had actually forgotten what "Old Dad" was like. We watched the "teenage years" DVD today. It featured Mom and "Old Dad." It was heartwarming to see the confident man that was sharp as a tack, and full of life and love, with a sparkle in his eyes once again. I am sure I will be watching these DVDs for the rest of my life and I will cherish them every time I do.

If you have parents that are still alive and in good mental condition, I strongly urge you to take the time to interview them, and capture it on a video. If you have children of your own, I strongly urge you to have someone interview you for them. It might even be a heartwarming gift to make an annual video of an interview with your children every year on their birthdays. Have them show you their favorite toys, what their favorite things to do are, show their room, ask them about their teachers and friends. What an incredible gift that would be to give them a compilation of all of those years.

Technology is a lot of fun to talk about and is quite fascinating to hear about, especially years from now. Tell them about your rotary phones and what it was like to only have a few channels on the TV and the days before remote controls when you actually had to turn the dial. Uh-oh, I'm dating myself here. They will be amazed to find out that a show was only shown once and that was it. If you missed it, you couldn't watch it again any time you wanted to. If you were lucky it would come on one more time in a rerun many months later. Seriously, though, those are the stories that will amaze your grandchildren some day, especially if you can show pictures of those items. Google them and print them out to show if you don't have pictures of your own. You'll have a great experience telling those stories, too. Who knows? Maybe they will even help *you* some day!

For those of you that still have fathers that are alive, give them a big hug and tell them you love them. Happy Father's Day! Oh! I almost forgot. Steve and I could actually understand all of what was said on the DVD without captions. That was one worry that we had when we were making the DVDs. We weren't sure we would actually be able to understand it later on. But with our CIs, we can.

July 6, 2014 HLAA Convention 2014 Austin, TX

I just attended my very first Hearing Loss Association of America convention. It was held in Austin, TX. I had a blast! It was truly remarkable that every single class and event were looped, and every word that was spoken was captioned for all to read. It was awesome. Even the music was looped. I learned a bit about loop systems and the T-Coil. I sure wish I had known about that when I wore my hearing aids. In case you don't know, a room can be "looped" by installing wires all around the room. Those wires transmit sound via a telecoil or T-Coil in a hearing device. Basically, the sound goes straight into the ears of the listener. It's kind of like a normal hearing person wearing headphones. These loop systems are usually installed in places like performing arts centers and public rooms but you can even loop your own home. I will be adding a T-Coil program as soon as I see my audiologist again so that I can hear better at the Orange County Performing Arts Center.

I think what I enjoyed the most was getting to spend time with so many different friends. Every meal was shared with someone different. I had met some of the people in person before and some I had only met through Facebook, chats, or forums. To meet them all face-to-face and get to converse with them in person was truly special.

One evening was a banquet and the entertainer was hard-of-hearing comedienne, Gael Hannan. The great thing was that the entire performance was captioned so I didn't miss a single word. She was *hilarious.* I laughed so hard I had tears pouring down my face and I could hardly breathe at one point. She did all deaf jokes, which every person in that room could relate to. She called us all "HOHs" at one point. I think it's safe to say there wasn't a dry eye in that place. My cheeks hurt I laughed so hard. HOH stands for hard-of-hearing, by the way.

They had a great Exhibit Hall. There were many, many vendors there. I sure wish I had known about HLAA when I had my hearing aids. There were so many devices I could have used then. I have no need for most of them now that I have my CIs. They had so many different listening devices. I did get a travel size alarm clock for the deaf. I think that will help when I go to Europe later this year. They even have doorbells, smoke alarms, and service dogs for deaf people. There was so much to see there.

I visited the Advanced Bionics booth. I was able to see the new Aqua Case accessory for the Naida processor. I also got to see the Phonak Roger Pen. I wasn't working the booth but, as soon as I arrived, I was asked if I would talk to someone that was thinking about getting a CI. I was more than happy to do that.

The classes were very good. There were so many different classes going on that it was impossible to attend each one. Some were geared towards hearing aid users, some for CI users, some were from vendors talking about their products, some were on relationships and communication, and some were on advocacy and employment issues. I even went to a class on identity theft. I'm not quite sure why they were there but it was good.

I attended a class on "Traveling the Globe with Hearing Loss and Cochlear Implants." I travel a lot, but I even learned something new. I didn't realize that you could check a "deaf" box when you buy a plane ticket and they will let you board early. Sometimes I can understand when they call my row but sometimes it's too noisy and I have to keep asking who is boarding. When I travel alone I think I will be checking that box. I did try that out when I flew home and it was kind of nice to get on first. They even put my bag in the overhead bin for me. I was also reminded about how electricity works in some foreign hotels. I will definitely use the tip I learned about that when I go overseas.

I took classes on enjoying music with a CI and an advocacy class. I will do my part to educate some local audiologists. I really enjoyed the Phonak presentation on the Roger pen. It looks like a regular pen but it is actually a microphone that is used in a variety of ways. It streams directly to a hearing aid or CI like wearing headphones would do. You can use it for one person speaking or for a table of people speaking. You can also use it to stream the TV and other devices like iPads, iPhones, etc. I am hoping to have a presentation on the Roger pen at one of our socials sometime soon.

There was even a casting call for "The Bachelor" TV show that I'm a big fan of. That had nothing to do with the convention but it was held at our hotel. I talked to the show staff and saw a lot of the people that were applying. That was fun. Lots of really pretty women showed up and a few men. Some were "wannabes" and some could definitely make it on the show. I even got a free pen.

It was a great trip and I'm so glad I went. I was especially happy to meet my two convention buddies that joined me at the hip, Larry and Candace. Thank you for all of the laughs and good times. To all of the rest of you that I met along the way (you know who you are) I won't soon forget you. You made my trip a special one.

August 9, 2014 *Fantasia* Accompanied by the Pacific Symphony Orchestra

I have always wanted to see Disney's animated film, *Fantasia*. Tonight it finally happened. It was even more special than seeing it in on TV or even in a movie theater, though. For one thing, we were celebrating all three of my brothers' birthdays so it was a family affair. Secondly, we saw it at the Verizon Wireless Amphitheater accompanied by the Pacific Symphony Orchestra.

We started out having a nice picnic dinner on the theater grounds then it was on to the show. The lights went down and the conductor came out. I understood every word he said. Our seats were pretty high up so I definitely couldn't see him. It was a real treat to be able to understand him throughout the whole show. Honestly, I'm not sure I'm ever going to be able to get over that. I think that is always going to be a big "wow" for me. Then the film came on and the music started. Unfortunately, we were too high up to actually watch the musicians. I was able to hear them, though, and I thoroughly enjoyed it!

I have never been good at telling which instrument is playing, even when I had perfect hearing. There were a couple of segments that had me baffled. I was curious which instruments were making the sounds that I was hearing. Fortunately, someone in our group had binoculars and I was able to see where the sounds were coming from. It turns out it was flutes playing along with plucking from violins. Very cool!

Steve was along, too. Unfortunately, he was not able to understand what was being spoken. However, when I asked him how the sound was for him, he got a big smile on his face and gave me a big thumbs up. He was definitely enjoying it, too.

August 30, 2014 Fishing with UltraZoom

I went fishing with Bob today. I've only fished once before, about twenty years ago. We had to get up very, very early. It was about 4:15 am. Bob dropped me off at the check in point and he went to park the car. I went up to the counter and knew I needed two fishing licenses. I'm afraid I couldn't understand the guy very well and just did the "nod and smile" when I heard him say "two fishing licenses." The next thing I know my credit card is charged $80 and I get the fishing licenses. He then brings out two fishing poles. Uh, wait a minute. I didn't order those. He said I said yes when he asked me. Oops! So back went the fishing poles and, evidently, the other things I said yes to. Back goes the credit card with $55 taken off. I'm going to chalk that one up to just being up too darned early in the morning.

We get on the boat and Bob informs me the very best spot is the very back center of the boat so we rush to get the prime spot. That also happens to be where the motor is and it is *loud*. On goes UltraZoom right away. Aaaaahhhh. Wonderful. UltraZoom consists of certain processor microphones that allow you to hear the person in front of you louder in noisy situations. This was the perfect setting to see just what it does. When I faced forward with the engine and wake crashing behind me, those sounds were very soft. When I turned my head to the side, those sounds got a little bit louder, which makes sense because if you are sitting at a table in a restaurant, for example, you want to be able to hear the person in front of you and next to you. When I faced the ocean, that noise was loud. I figured out that the best way to have a conversation was with the ocean behind me.

I have to admit that I was secretly pleased with my superpowers. I was able to understand Bob in his regular voice but he had to keep asking me to repeat what I was saying with my regular voice. He did better listening to the announcements though. I wasn't able to understand what the captain was saying through the loudspeaker very well.

UltraZoom definitely saved the day for me as I was able to talk to other people on the boat easily, too. I wish I had been awake when I talked to the guy at the check in, as I would have realized I should have switched to UltraZoom there, too.

By the way, I caught seven fish. And . . . it will probably be another twenty years before I do that again!

September 14, 2014 Elvis is Still The King

I have a love/hate relationship with music with my cochlear implants. I hate that the singers don't sound the way I remember them. I love that I can understand some lyrics in songs, even in songs I have never heard before.

I had a "wow" moment on my way home tonight. I was listening to an oldies station and clearly heard Elvis Presley's voice just the way I remembered him. It wasn't a song that I was familiar with but I knew immediately it was Elvis. When I got home I Googled the song, *Little Sister,* just to see if it really was Elvis singing and it was. I understood some of the lyrics, too, which always puts a smile on my face.

It is times like these that give me hope that maybe someday the "hate" will go out of my relationship with music.

September 28, 2014 Jury Duty Summons

I received a jury duty summons the other day. For the first time ever I was actually excited to get it. When I was a kid I wanted to be a trial lawyer. I loved debating and giving speeches. When I started losing my hearing, I gave up on that idea. I wanted to be the best and was worried that I would miss something important that was said in the courtroom.

Whenever I was called to jury duty, I would get a bit of anxiety. I was afraid I'd say something stupid to the judge like giving the answer to a question I thought he asked, but actually being asked a completely different question. If you've got a hearing loss you probably know exactly what I just said. The rest of you are probably scratching your heads. I was also worried that I would miss vital testimony and that I would miss things that were said with the other jurors when making a decision. Deciding someone's fate in a courtroom is serious business and I was worried that I would screw it up by making a decision based on wrong information.

In the olden days, I was able to give my lack of hearing as an excuse and I wouldn't have to go at all. Then technology got better and they provided CART. That is where they have someone sit with you all day that has a laptop. They type everything that is said. I used that one time and it was pretty nice. Another time I went, but they forgot to schedule the CART person so I was excused after only an hour.

I've never actually made it out of the jury room into a courtroom. I've actually been happy to have my handicap in the past because I worked full time and didn't get paid for my jury service. I didn't really want to be there. Now I work part time and I can hear. I'm not going to ask for CART assistance this time because I really do think I can do it on my own. For the first time ever, I'm actually hoping I get on a jury. I'll let you know if I do!

October 22, 2014 Mediterranean Vacation

I just returned from an incredible two week vacation. My mom and I went on a land tour of Croatia and Slovenia for the first week. We went on a Mediterranean cruise to Venice, Italy; Dubrovnik, Croatia; Ephesus, Turkey; Santorini, Greece; and Olympia, Greece for the second week. Having cochlear implants on this trip made it very easy. I was able to do a lot of things that I couldn't do on trips like this in the past with my hearing aids.

As always, flights are best with a hearing loss. There is a lot of noise from the engine. If I wanted it quiet, I simply took my processors off. I slept and read in complete silence. My poor mother was not so lucky. Now if I could only do something to stop the kid behind me from hitting my seat every few minutes.

I brought a couple of different battery types with me. I brought my Zinc Air disposable batteries for the plane ride. I knew it was going to be a really long time from when we left home until we arrived in Croatia and I didn't want to have to deal with changing batteries. I also wasn't sure how the electrical outlets were going to be at the European hotels. At one hotel I couldn't find any outlets so having the Zinc Air batteries gave me peace of mind. I used my regular rechargeable batteries most of the time, though. I do have a duplicate set so one set was always charged and ready to go even if I couldn't charge overnight. We stayed at different hotels every night on our land tour, by the way.

Our land tour consisted of my mother, Jakov (our tour guide), and me. Jakov drove us everywhere and I sat in the front passenger seat. Jakov is a history buff and he filled us with information everywhere we went. It was heavenly to actually be able to look out and enjoy the sights and still be able to understand what he was saying in the car. We drove a lot on the trip and we talked pretty much the whole time. With hearing aids, I would have had to look at Jakov the entire time in order to read his lips to understand what he was saying.

We took different tours at every port when we were on the cruise. One tour was with a large group. We went on what looked like a pirate ship. Our guide gave us a device with earbuds and she spoke to us through that. With my Naida processor, I have T-Mics. These are microphones that sit at the opening of the ear canal. I was very grateful to have this type of microphone because I was easily able to use the earbuds and I could understand some of what she was saying. I say "some" because she had a fairly whiney voice that I didn't like very much and I tuned her out a lot.

I took a self-guided tour of Ephesus in Turkey. Again, they gave us iPods with earbuds. We were given an hour and a half to walk through and see whatever we could during that time. The iPod had tracks with each point of interest along with directions on where to go to get to the next point of interest. I understood everything that was said on that tour. It was great!

We took a special tour when we were in Santorini, Greece. The tour guide was a professional photographer. He gave me a photography class teaching me many different things about my camera. He also took us to some incredible spots on the island where I experimented with what he taught me. Again, it was nice not to have to read his lips while he was showing me the different features on my camera. I was able to watch what he was doing while listening at the same time. I didn't miss a thing and I understood exactly what he was telling me. And I got some great pictures.

We went to many shows and activities on the cruise. I was able to easily understand all of the shows no matter where we sat in the room. I participated in the music trivia every night and could easily hear the music. I even won a ton of logo merchandise in the "What are the Lyrics?" game show. They would play part of a song then you had to go up to the microphone and sing the rest of it.

It was so nice being a normal hearing person on this entire trip. I don't think I uttered the dreaded four letter word, "What?", more than a couple of times. It's truly been a fantastic experience, and I am so grateful for the miracle of my cochlear implants!

November 22, 2014 Juror #10!

I told you before how excited I was to get my jury summons. Well, I called in on Friday, November 14th after 5:00 pm, and out of seventeen groups, only two groups were called to report to the courthouse on Monday morning. You guessed it. I was one of them. In the olden days that would have really made me mad. But now that I can actually hear, I got a bit excited.

I got to the jury assembly room and picked my seat. I chose the second row back in the center right by the podium and screen. Some habits are just hard to break. You see, I've been sitting in seats similar to that for thirty years because it's the best place to read lips. Of course, now I can sit anywhere in the room, but sometimes that anxiety is still there when I am back in a situation that caused anxiety in the past. I looked around the room and saw that there were very few people there. I figured we had a pretty good chance of making it into a courtroom. The next thing I knew there was someone speaking on the loudspeaker. They didn't come out to the podium, and I understood every word. She talked for a little while and then instructed the entire room to report to courtroom sixteen. I actually got up at the same time as everyone else did and knew exactly where we were going. For those of you that aren't hearing impaired, I'm sure you are wondering why that is a "wow" moment for me. Those of you with hearing loss are probably cheering. I definitely would have been lost before, and would have had to have asked someone what was said and where we were going.

I took my seat in courtroom sixteen. The dreaded roll call was next. I listened very carefully, wanting to make sure I didn't miss my name. I noticed that the names were being called alphabetically. After intently listening through the D's, I realized that I understood every single name that was called very easily and I relaxed a bit. "Julie Husting?" "Here!" Piece of cake!

Then it came time for them to call the names of the prospective jurors and alternates. My name was called tenth. There were eighteen names called altogether. They had each of us give answers to about six questions. The questions were written out for everyone to see. There was a row of people behind me and another row of people in front of me. I was curious to see how much of that I would get. There were different accents with Vietnamese and Latino among them. Some people spoke very quietly. The judge was actually the worst one of all. His voice was *very* deep. It didn't help that I was not able to see his lips at all from my vantage point. I understood most of what people were saying, including the judge. I'm pretty sure that the ones I couldn't understand nobody else could either. In fact, the judge even asked some people to repeat what they said because he couldn't understand either. The funny thing is that I found myself interpreting what the judge was saying to two of the prospective jurors.

One by one people were being questioned and excused from serving on a jury . . . except for me. They didn't ask me any questions, and I wasn't excused. More and more prospective jurors filled the empty seats and the questions and answers began again and more people were excused. It was pretty clear I was to be "Juror #10."

Jury selection finally ended in the afternoon and the trial began. It was a driving under the influence (DUI) case. Both attorneys gave their opening statements and then we heard from the first witness who was the arresting officer. The courtroom was very quiet and I was easily able to understand everything that was said. I kept my poker face on for the court, but I was beaming inside.

We reconvened on Tuesday and listened to two more witnesses. It became more and more clear that the defendant was guilty as charged. I have no idea why he even decided to pay a lawyer to go to court. The lawyer was grasping at straws at his ridiculous defense. It was hard for me not to yell out, "Really? That's the best you can come up with?" Even he knew he had no case.

After a two hour lunch we listened to the closing arguments. Then we went to deliberate. Once again, twelve people around a conference room gave me a little bit of anxiety. You see, we used to have weekly management meetings where we sat around a similar conference table. I used to have to really concentrate in those meetings and had a hard time understanding people at the other end of the table. I made sure to sit in the center of the long table, just in case. As usual, I need not have worried. I understood everyone just fine. It turns out that I didn't need to understand them for very long because it took all of thirty seconds for each of us to declare the defendant guilty.

It was my pleasure to get a drunk driver off the streets!

January 4, 2015 My Amazing Mom

I recently told you about a great vacation I took with my mom, Midge Husting. Before we went on that trip, my mom had a growth in her gums. We were under the impression it was some kind of gum disease. She had her tooth pulled when we got home as well as that growth. It turns out that growth was actually a malignant tumor. Our lives have been turned upside down for the past couple of months. It's not every day you hear the dreaded "C" word.

Mom had surgery on December 1st to remove half of her lower jawbone. The cancer was in there as well as some lymph nodes. I moved in with her when she got out of the hospital and have been there ever since. I will likely go back home soon. She was told she needed radiation. But, after hearing how horrible it is and what her life would be like afterwards, as well as no guarantee that the cancer still wouldn't come back, she's decided not to have it. I can't say that I blame her.

That's what's been happening in my life for the past couple of months. What I really wanted to tell you about is what an amazing woman my mother is. People often mention what a positive person I am, how even in hard times, I try to see the bright side of the situation. I get that attitude from my mom. I completely fell apart when she told me she had cancer. But not Mom. She seemed completely unfazed by it. I had asked her if she was worried and she just said that she had lived a very eventful, full, happy life and if it was her time to go then it was her time. She said there was nothing she could do about it, so why worry? I grabbed ahold of her strength and took her cue. I don't think I cried again until we met with the radiation team of doctors. They were pretty brutal and we both had a good cry after seeing them. Other than that, we simply took each day and each doctor's appointment as it came.

They were able to get all of her cancer out. She was told there was a 60% chance of the cancer coming back if she didn't have radiation. She has decided not to worry about that either. She is determined to be in the 40% with the people that the cancer never comes back. Someone has to make up that percentage so it may as well be her. Our plan is to continue to live life to its fullest just as she has been. If the cancer does come back, we will deal with it then. But in the meantime, look out world! We've got places to go and things to do!

I have learned from her that a good attitude will get you a happy life. I have no doubt that there are two kinds of people in this world. If people were told they had six months to live, there are those that would worry and count the days until they die and those that would make the most out of every day that they have left and would challenge that six months to be twelve. Mom falls in the latter category of people.

She has always taught me that I could do anything I wanted to do. I simply had to set my mind to it and get it done. I think that's why my hearing loss has never really been a negative issue in my life. She never felt sorry for me (at least not to my face) and so I never felt sorry for myself either. It simply was what it was, and I just had to make the most of it.

It's funny because we've never really been a "why me?" kind of family. I immediately thought of my dad, who passed away in March, when I found out my mom had cancer. I could just imagine him calling down, "Honey! I miss you! I want you here with me!" I immediately yelled back, "You can't have her, Dad! I'm not finished with her yet!" I promised him I would take good care of her and he could have her for eternity, but not yet. All in good time. Silly, I know, but it made the "reason" of "why her" a little easier to understand. A person could go crazy otherwise.

Another lesson she taught me that I will always be grateful for, was to never worry about what other people would think. That lesson has allowed me to just be me. If people like me, then that's great. If not, no big deal. I am who I am they can take it or leave it. It's very freeing to be that way. Mom and I have made complete fools of ourselves in public and boy, have we had fun doing it. She is a blast to be around because she is who she is and makes no apologies for it.

She is also the kindest, most giving person I know. Many people, including myself, gossip. I can't remember a time when she's ever said anything bad about anyone. She has always looked for the good in everyone and in every situation. She goes out of her way to help people. She is eighty-six years old and still teaches rubber stamping classes. She will go out of her way to do part of the projects to help the "old" people in her class. Amazing, I tell you! Even when she was told she was having surgery on December 1st, she insisted on finishing her weekly classes that were scheduled through Thanksgiving. She didn't want to let anyone down.

I know this chapter didn't have anything to do about my hearing and that's what this book is for. I will say this, though, we have been to countless doctors' appointments and I have been on the phone a *lot* in the past couple of months for her and I have understood every single thing. I have not struggled one single time with hearing. In this time of craziness, that is one thing I have been truly grateful for.

It is a new year, and life is getting back to normal now. Mom is back to eating real food again. She looks much more like her old self and has made tremendous improvement. Mom and I have a trip planned at the end of January to go to Orlando, Florida for the Stampin' Up! Leadership Conference. We also have a week long European cruise planned with the whole family in June. I'm sure there will be a lot more little mini trips and fun things to do the rest of the year as well. And beyond that, too!

 # Trip to Orlando, Florida

I just spent the week in sunny Orlando, Florida with my good friend, Glad, and my mom. It was time, once again, for the Stampin' Up! Leadership Conference. The great news was that my mom finally got to go with me again. She has not been able to attend for several years due to caring for my dad, who had Alzheimer's. The bad news is that this was the last Leadership Conference that Stampin' Up! will be having.

We had a free day on our first day. We went to Universal Studios. We went to the Harry Potter section first. I had a little bit of anxiety on some of the rides. I really wanted to be able to hear everything, but I was worried that my processors might fall off. Some of the rides were considered "thrill" rides but they were not your typical roller coaster style. I was especially worried on the first one because there was a harness that made it so that I couldn't cover my ears with my hands. That meant I couldn't hold onto my processors. It turns out that my processors were safe on that one, even though we twisted and turned and went almost upside down and shook quite a bit. I'm going to throw in a disclaimer here: I can't guarantee that your processor won't fall off. I was actually kicking myself that I didn't wear my Neptune processors instead of my Naidas. My Neptune processors are clipped on and they are connected to my headpiece and T-Mic by a wire so I would not have lost them even if they did come off my ear. We went on another ride that was similar to this one but it didn't have the shoulder harness. This time I look one of my processors off. I also kept my hand over my ear, just in case. The headpiece did come off once this time, but not the processor itself. I believe that was due to the 3D glasses I wore and where the arm was in relation to my cord. The processor stayed on my ear, though, so no harm done.

The rides themselves were really well done. I'm not a big Harry Potter fan but I really loved all of the rides and the scenery throughout the area. They had a very cool train ride that got us from Universal Studios to Islands of Adventure (another theme park). That train was also a ride with lots of things to see and hear along the way. In the queue to get onto one of the Harry Potter rides, Harry Potter and his friends came out and talked to the people in line. I was not able to understand what they said. The old guy that I'm assuming must be a headmaster (I know, I know, you Harry Potter fans are cringing) also came out and talked to us but I couldn't understand what he was saying either. They had painted portraits hanging in a gallery that we went by and those paintings came to life and talked to each other. I was able to understand those. Very cool.

I went on a regular roller coaster and definitely removed my ears for that one. We went on many other rides and saw some shows. I was able to understand good ol' Shrek and his friends, even though they are animated characters. Very fun day!

The next several days we were at the conference. I did not have any of the anxiety that I have had in the past. In fact, I did not even use the "special needs" perks that Stampin' Up! provides to those with hearing loss. Instead, I got in line with the rest of the demonstrators and I chose my seat based on how well I could see what was being shown to us, rather than what I needed to be able to see in order to hear. I understood probably 99% of what was said. In fact, it was *so* easy that I began to question whether or not I really did struggle in the past. Could my hearing really have changed that much?

After the conference was over, that question was answered. My old reflection was looking back at me in the form of my friend, Becky. I have sat with her in the special needs section at many Stampin' Up! events. She, too, has a profound hearing loss. I felt great sadness when she told me she could not understand the keynote speaker as he walked around the stage and turned his head away from her. I could also tell that she was not able to understand my mom as she spoke to her. My mom has what I call "bad lips" due to some swelling from her recent jaw surgery. When you have to read lips to "hear", bad lips are a disaster. I knew exactly how Becky was feeling and I felt so guilty when she asked how I was doing. I want so badly for her to be able to experience what I am. Unfortunately, she is not able to get a cochlear implant.

By watching Becky interact with my mom, it made me so very grateful that I got my CIs when I did. It would have made caring for her after her cancer surgery extremely difficult if I would have had to read her lips to understand her. It was already a very difficult situation and that would have made it so much worse. I'm extremely lucky.

Back to the conference — the keynote speaker, Jason Wright, was fantastic. He talked about the power of a handwritten letter. In this day and age of social media and email, handwritten letters are a rarity. I have to wonder if the younger generation has ever written or received one. His speech made us laugh and cry. I could tell I was not the only one crying as I heard all of the people sniffling all around me. I'm going to throw a challenge out to all of you that are reading this: send a hand written letter to someone that has made an impact on your life and tell them how much they mean to you. It could be your parent, your child, another relative, a best friend, a teacher, or anyone. They will likely keep it and may need it to comfort them if you should pass away before they do. In fact, I was recently shown two letters that I had written to two different people many years ago. They had kept my letters and it was pretty neat to read them again. I had forgotten some of the memories that I had shared and it was nice to relive those moments.

On our last night we went to BB Kings Blues Club for dinner. The food was great and a live band started playing just after we finished dinner. Fortunately, I have the UltraZoom feature on my processor. That feature makes the sound that is in front of me louder and lessens sounds that are around me. I could easily hear the band, but I was also fairly easily able to understand my mom and Glad when they talked. They, on the other hand, were having a hard time hearing each other because the music was *so* loud. I was actually the one with the advantage in hearing. I experimented with the music on my different programs and it sounded great no matter which program I had on.

It was a really great trip and I am so fortunate to be blessed by this miracle called a cochlear implant. I'm also so grateful to have my mom going to Stampin' Up! events with me again.

March 28, 2015 Patience Pays Off for Steve

A question I'm often asked is how long it took until I could understand easily with my CIs and didn't have to read lips anymore. I really hate to answer that question because everyone is different and it isn't a race. If you've read this far, you know that it came fairly quickly for me but that is not typically the case with most people. A lot of different factors determine when it will happen: your "hearing history" (how long you could hear normally before you lost your hearing), your age, how much rehab you do, how much you wear your CI by itself, how much you wear your CI each day, how much you are actually listening to something (ie; not alone in a quiet house), and just plain dumb luck.

It has been two years since Steve had his first CI. I have lunch with Steve every week. We also work for the same company but in different departments. Just in this last month, I have seen great improvements. In fact, even one of his co-workers came to me and told me what a miracle it is. Steve's desk is in a bullpen area and his co-worker is in an office next to his. She told me she was whistling and he asked (from the other room) if anyone was whistling. She said it was her and asked, "Could you hear that, Steve?" and he answered her. (okay, now I'm getting emotional just writing this!) Words just can't describe how big that seemingly simple exchange really is. This is the same guy who, I can't tell you how many times, I have stood just a few feet from him and called his name and he never turned around. Now he can understand his co-worker in another room.

We go to lunch with my other brother, Curtis, and another co-worker every Friday. It used to be that Steve could barely understand me sitting with him in the backseat. Just recently, I have noticed that he is now talking to Curtis, who is driving, with Steve sitting behind him in the backseat. He is not reading his lips nor is he straining to understand what is being said. (Dang! Where's the Kleenex?) I can't tell you how *thrilled* I am to witness this. It truly is a miracle.

Remember, this is two years later that these changes are happening. He had a mapping recently and told me what his comprehension is now. I can't remember what the actual score was, but I know that it was a great improvement from when he was tested the previous time. He still has room to grow and I'm confident that he is going to continue to evolve. The point I'm trying to make here is that, you can't give up. Our ears continue to evolve even two years later. I see people get discouraged that they are still reading lips six months after their first CI. Whenever that happens, I ask them what they *can* do now that they couldn't do with hearing aids and I usually get a pretty long list.

I always encourage people to start a hearing journal, which is simply a daily log that lists what new things they heard that day, as well as things they are still having a hard time with. There are days that can be very frustrating when you feel like you're not making any progress. It is on those days, that I encourage people to take out the journal and read it. When you can see all of the things that you can do now that you couldn't do before, right there in black and white, it is very encouraging. It is also nice to read all of the things that you couldn't do in the early stages and see that you can do them now.

The three P's are *extremely* important in this journey: Practice, Persistence and, most of all, Patience! Some people even add Prayer. Don't give up! Life is good.

May 11, 015 # Phantom Sounds

Hopefully, you've read some of this book already and know that I am fairly sane. Once you read this chapter, you might question my sanity. Before I had my CIs and I wore hearing aids, I could hear myself talk even when my hearing aids were out. I couldn't hear anyone else but I could hear myself. When I had talked to my surgeon about what would happen after I had the CI surgery, he told me that I would be completely deaf. I asked him if I would still hear myself talk when I wasn't wearing my processors. He said, "Uh, no . . . I just told you. You are going to be completely deaf." I was a bit worried about going *completely* deaf.

I remember thinking about it a lot and wondering if I was *really* hearing myself talk when I wasn't wearing my hearing aids. After all, I couldn't hear anybody else and the only other sound I heard was the horrendous clanging of tinnitus. I had a tiny bit of residual hearing but I could only hear someone if they yelled directly into my ears. Obviously, I wasn't talking while someone was doing that.

I went ahead with the surgery but was worried about hearing absolute complete silence. I was quite relieved when I *could* still hear myself talk, even without my processors on. It is much quieter because I don't have the horrendous tinnitus any more but it is far from silent. Now I hear what I would call white noise. Surprisingly, I also hear a lot more than my own voice. When I'm brushing my teeth, I hear the water running, the sounds of the toothbrush on my teeth, and the splash when I spit out the water. I also hear my steps when I walk, the water run when I am in the shower, and I pretty much hear other sounds that I can see, too.

I am not *really* hearing these sounds, as I really am completely deaf when I am not wearing my processors. I call these "phantom sounds." My brain is filling in the gaps of what my ears (bionic or not) are not hearing. It knows what those sounds are, as my eyes can see them, and I can even feel the vibrations in some cases. If someone is behind me making sounds then I can't hear them, as my brain doesn't know those sounds are happening.

I've heard about people that no longer have limbs that they once had and how they can still feel them there. I imagine this is a similar sensation to that.

Whenever I hear new CI candidates who are terrified of losing their residual hearing, I have to wonder if what they are really worried about is losing the phantom sounds that they are hearing. Because let's face it, if you qualify for a CI, you aren't really hearing much without your hearing aids on. Now, Advanced Bionics has a different electrode that does preserve some residual hearing but that came out after I was implanted.

I have no idea of there is a real term for "phantom sounds" and have only discussed this with a few of my CI friends once. I just know that I am grateful for them and that my world isn't completely silent when my ears aren't turned on.

July 1, 2015 Unexpected Side Effect

Before I got my cochlear implants, I knew exactly one person with a hearing loss. Steve. Then I began doing research on CIs and I came across hearingjourney.com. It is Advanced Bionics' forum where CI users help each other out.

Through this forum I met Cindy, who was having her first surgery on the same day I was having mine. We sent daily emails talking about our experience. She then introduced me to a very small group that was working on rehab exercises via email every day. It was there that I met Paul, Larry, Rose, Kirsten, and several others. We became a pretty tight knit group that chats daily to this day. Last month, we had a reunion in Washington State and spent a whole week together. It was awesome!

I became a mentor soon after getting my first CI and I met many more tremendous people. I met them individually when they were referred to me and others I have met through our Bionic Ear Association social gatherings that we have quarterly. I cherish many of these friendships that I have made. If you are in Southern California and have an Advanced Bionics CI or are thinking about getting a CI, we would love to have you join us at our socials. See the Afterward for my contact information.

I also went on a retreat through Advanced Bionics to meet other mentors. My friendships grew across the country and I had a fantastic time getting together with them at the hearing loss convention last year, where I made even more friends.

When I began looking into getting a cochlear implant, I simply wanted to be able to understand speech again. I never ever expected it to change my life by rewarding me with such close friendships. I love watching new friendships blossom online and at our socials. It's truly one of the best side effects I've ever seen!

September 27, 2015 Update on Steve

I was at the office on Friday. Steve came in and sat down in front of me. One of our co-workers sits at her desk next to me. Between us is a row of filing cabinets. She joined in our conversation and Steve understood everything she was saying and responded to her very easily. I was shocked. If I hadn't seen it with my own eyes, I'm not sure I would have believed it. Just then, another co-worker came by. I told him what I just witnessed and he said that he and Steve have conversations across the room all the time. Wow! This is *huge* progress. I remember the days when we could stand right behind him and yell his name and he wouldn't turn around. We always had to tap him on the back or stand in front of him to get his attention.

He is getting really good at understanding from the back seat of the car, too. He is understanding what the people in the front seat say, too. We talked about music at lunchtime. He had mentioned a few months back that music was too noisy. I asked him what he was listening to and he said pop music. I recommended that he try "easy listening" on Pandora. He's tried it and he really likes it. He especially likes Michael Bublé and Harry Connick Jr. He is even understanding some of the lyrics now. Steve hasn't listened to music since he was around twenty, about thirty years ago. Again, this is really spectacular progress. I can't tell you how happy I am for him!

It should be noted that he got his CI over two and a half years ago. Progress is still being made. Many people with CIs get discouraged if they are still reading lips after three months. The reality is that it takes time. If you think about it, though, two and a half years is a very short period of time when you consider that Steve has had his hearing loss for fifty years. When you consider how many years he has left to live, a couple of years is just a blip!

December 26, 2015 *Star Wars*

There's this little movie that seems to have taken the world by storm. Perhaps you've heard of it. It's called, *Star Wars: The Force Awakens*. If you have a CI and are a *Star Wars* fan and you haven't been to a movie since your hearing aid days, then it's time to get to the theater.

For many of us, going to the movies probably brings up fond and bad memories at the same time. Maybe you recall going to the movies when your hearing was still good. I had perfect hearing when I saw the first *Star Wars* movie many years ago. If memory serves me correctly, I believe I saw it many times back then. I went to the movies regularly for a long time. Then my hearing got worse and I was missing too much of what was said and I stopped going. Seeing movies on the small TV screen and understanding the words, beats seeing it on the big screen and not understanding it. I imagine that is the same for many of you that have cochlear implants.

I know you likely still use your captions on your TV and they likely didn't have captions at the movies the last time you went. Well, most theaters do now. I, too, still use the captions on my TV and I do get the captioning device when I go to the movies. Do I rely on them when I'm at the movies? Not always, but it's a nice security blanket to have in case I need it. I have gone back to going to the movies regularly now and I enjoy it as much as I used to when I had good hearing.

I saw the new *Star Wars* movie and loved it. I understood everything. I can't tell you what percentage I used the captions as I really wasn't conscious of it. I probably used them a lot because I didn't want to take the chance of missing anything. I simply put the cupholder device with a little captioning screen directly underneath the big screen and it's very easy to read and still enjoy the movie. Some theaters use glasses that have captions on them.

My brother, Steve, saw it, too. He went on opening night. His captioning device wasn't working perfectly, but he did understand it, even when the captions weren't working. He was even thrilled to find out he could understand the creature characters without the device. He saw it a second time and was able to get the entire movie that time.

If that doesn't convince you, remember, it's good rehab practice. The worst that can happen is you get to see an awesome movie and enjoy a great visual experience and then you can follow it up at home on DVD to catch anything you may have missed. Be sure to see it in 3D.

January 9, 2016 Music Breakthrough

I think it's finally happened! Vocals are finally starting to sound just as I remember them. This is *huge*.

As you know, I have a love/hate relationship with my cochlear implants and music. I've loved listening to music since I was a little girl. Hearing aids amplify what your ears can hear. If your ears are damaged then the sound quality probably isn't clear but they still hear regular voices and music. However, when I got to the profound hearing loss stage, I was having a hard time listening to music in my car. I couldn't hear it over the other noises and it was taking me longer and longer to figure out which songs I was hearing. Forget about trying to make out any words on new songs or songs I didn't know by heart. That never happened with my hearing aids. But when I listened on my computer at home, music still sounded the way I'd heard it growing up.

Everything changed, musically, when I got my cochlear implants. When I was first activated, any songs that I didn't know sounded like screeching cats. It was horrendous. Songs I did know sounded like the munchkins re-recorded all of my music. Fortunately, that is normal in the very, very early stages of getting switched on. That doesn't last long. Within a short period of time, instruments sound fairly normal but, for some reason, vocals don't. For me, most of the vocals sounded like the same person was singing every song. Female vocalists, especially, all sounded the same.

I had a bit of a panic attack when I went to a Styx concert in the early stages of my CI. It was like watching a cover band of one of my favorite groups. I was really, really afraid of someday forgetting what they actually sounded like. That's where a good hearing history comes in. Memory helps your brain fill in the blanks to reconcile what you are actually hearing versus what your mind knows it should be.

Since receiving cochlear implants, I've still been enjoying music tremendously. I can pretty much immediately recognize songs I know. I can often understand a lot of lyrics being sung, even on songs I don't know. I have developed a love for country music because the lyrics are often easier to understand than pop and rock music. Although, I still love those genres as well. I love listening to music in my car again.

The other day, while I was working, I was listening to my old music on iTunes. I soon realized that Mick Jagger sounded like Mick Jagger. Shania Twain was Shania. Could it be? Yes! Freddie Mercury and Elton John were themselves. This was a really big breakthrough. Here comes Steve Perry. That voice. It's definitely him. It seems that I've got my men back and Shania. I will need to listen to my other favorite female singers and see how they rate now compared to how I remember them.

My friend, David, kept telling me to hang in there. That voices would come back to me and he was so right. It's taken several years but it is finally happening!

January 10, 2016 Perfect Evening at a Concert

If you read the last chapter, you know that vocals are finally sounding "right" to me again. As it turns out, it couldn't have come at a better time. A friend, Chaz, had invited me to the Donny Osmond concert a while back. Forgetting that I had a disappointing concert experience and had vowed not to go to concerts anymore, I said yes. Well, now I'm sure glad I did. But I'm getting too far ahead of myself.

First, we had about a twenty-five minute drive to my favorite restaurant, Stacked. I hadn't seen Chaz in a really long time, and he had quite a bit of news to catch me up on. He talked quite a bit in the car ride. In the dark, I might add. In my hearing aid days, this would have been a disaster. Those days are far gone and I thoroughly enjoyed listening to him while I was driving. I understood every word and didn't need to ask him to repeat a thing.

The restaurant was pretty noisy but it was no problem for me. I switched to my UltraZoom program. We had a great conversation with super yummy food.

Then we got to the performing arts center. We got our tickets a bit late so the best seats available at the time were on the fifth level, which was the farthest up and back that you could get. Forget trying to see Donny's face let alone his lips. There was no giant screen to see him "live" either. He started singing and, at first, the sound wasn't that great. I decided to switch to my UltraZoom program since all of the speakers were in front of us. That worked great. I got all of the instruments and he came through loud and clear. The best part of all was that it was *him* singing. It was really his voice I was hearing. He sang a few of his old songs and many more new songs that I hadn't heard him sing. His voice was definitely what I heard on every song. There was no cover band here.

He told stories almost as much as he sang and I could easily understand every word he said, too. Again, this would have been completely unheard of in my hearing aid days. I would have been totally lost and frustrated through most of it.

We had a very nice drive home with great conversation. It was a perfectly "normal" evening. Sometimes I think I will just take this all for granted but several times during the night I would think to myself, "I'm really getting this! Wow!" I don't think it ever gets old. I am truly blessed.

June 16, 2016 Another Wish List Item Checked Off

One of the first things I tell people that are getting a cochlear implant is to make up a Wish List of things they can no longer hear that they hope to hear again some day with their cochlear implant. It's been three and a half years and I can finally check off yet another item from my list.

I was hiking with a friend yesterday and I was telling her about my wish list. One of the items I checked off right away was to hear birds. I told her about hiking with a friend when I still had hearing aids and I asked her if she could hear any birds. She said she could and proceeded to tell me where they were and how many there were. I was amazed that she could do that. Now, of course, I almost take it for granted, just as my hearing friend did until I told her about it. She promptly closed her eyes and just listened to everything she could hear. Then she admitted that, yes, she didn't even give those sounds a second thought.

Three miles later we were hiking down a very steep hill. All of a sudden I heard someone calling out and the sound of a bike coming. I immediately jumped to the right, out of harm's way. Boy, was I glad I heard him, because he was coming *fast*. Sure enough, just a few minutes later, I heard another bike coming and I got out of the way. That was one of the few items I had left to cross off my wish list. Normally, whoever I was hiking with has to yank me out of the way or tell me to move over. I'm glad I did it myself this time because my friend did not tell me. I think she's used to me hearing now.

For some reason, the sound of bike tires has eluded me until now. I think because it is so faint. I only have a couple of items left to check off on my wish list. I'm sure they will be checked off some day.

We saw a tree growing between two big boulders on our hike. It kind of reminded me of my hearing being set free and blooming after being locked in for so long.

November 24, 2016 # I am Truly Grateful

I had to take a minute, on this day of Thanksgiving, to thank Advanced Bionics for the incredible gift they have given me. I just passed my four year anniversary of my first cochlear implant (my second one was six months later). I am still amazed at everything that I can do now that I couldn't do before.

I was recently at Advanced Bionics as a research subject. One day I had to listen to sentences and repeat back what I was hearing. I could understand almost 100% in the quiet setting. It was so easy and I didn't have to concentrate. I did really well when they added noise, too. It took more concentration but I did it. It still amazes me that I can do this without reading lips.

I then worked with two gentlemen that were talking among themselves. I only had one of my CIs on for most of the time. I purposely looked down to see how much I could understand. Sometimes their voices were low as they were just quietly trying things. I'm glad they weren't paying any attention to me because they would notice that I had a pretty big grin on my face. I could clearly understand everything they were saying even though sometimes their voices were barely above a whisper.

I love listening to music on my car radio. Now that singers' voices sound normal again, it is very enjoyable listening to my old music. I still get quite a kick out of listening to new music and understanding some lyrics. Shoot, just the fact that I can listen to music on the radio in my car is a feat in itself!

I love hearing the front door unlock in the other room when my man comes home in the evening. I can also hear the floor above me creak when I'm downstairs and I know that he's awake. I can hear my cat's bell tinkling and I know that she has entered the room and is near. She talks to me a lot now. She didn't do that as much when I had hearing aids. I'm guessing she figured out that I didn't hear her as much.

I think my co-workers get a kick out of being able to call my name after I've passed by their office and I turn around and go back. I love that I can call out to another co-worker clear across the room and I can ask him a question and get an answer without even seeing him.

I enjoy going out to dinner with my friends, even a group of friends. I can understand the various conversations going on and can actually participate in them without worrying that I'm going to say something that doesn't pertain to the conversation because I heard it wrong.

Driving with a passenger is so much more enjoyable. I can carry on a conversation without having to try to drive and read lips at the same time. It doesn't even matter if it's dark. I can be a passenger in the back seat and talk to the other passengers in the front seat, too.

On most days I take my good hearing for granted. But every now and then it hits me what is happening and just how far I've come.

December 5, 2016 The Best Gift You Can Give: A Message to the Hearing Community

Well, the *best* gift is probably diamonds! But, seriously, if you want to give a gift that will be treasured every day for the rest of their life, banish the words "never mind" from your vocabulary, especially if you have a friend or loved one that has hearing loss. Imagine this simple conversation between a person with normal hearing and a person that is hearing impaired:

"It's cold outside."

"What?"

"Never mind."

When the hearing person says, "Never mind" they are thinking, "Oh, it's just small talk. It's not important." But what the hearing impaired person hears is, "*You* are not important. You are not worth my time in repeating what I said."

Really think about this for a second. How much of what is said on a daily basis really *is* important? Small talk pretty much makes up the majority of conversations. None of them are really important. In fact, we likely forget the majority of what we hear within a few hours of hearing it. I bet you're thinking about that now, too. Go ahead — what was the conversation you had with someone four hours ago? Do you remember? What did you talk about yesterday? Shoot, I can't even remember what I was wearing yesterday.

What small talk does, though, is gives us a connection to others. It gives meaning and context to our relationships. It says, "I like you. I want to share a moment with you. You matter to me." When you take it back by saying "never mind" you are saying just the opposite. Those words are extremely hurtful to those with hearing loss. You have to realize that people with hearing aids typically have to concentrate very hard on what you are saying. They likely have to read your lips, read your facial cues and study the tone of your voice. It takes a lot of effort on their part to understand you. What effort are you making?

The best gift that you can give is to make an effort. Speak slowly. Speak loudly if that's what your loved one needs. Yes, it's embarrassing to talk loudly in public. Yes, people will hear what you are saying. Do it anyway. Don't talk while you're chewing. Don't cover your mouth when you're speaking. Look at them. Make the effort.

Let your loved one speak for themselves when talking to others, too. I am a mentor. One of the things I do is meet with people that are thinking about getting cochlear implants or with people that may be having problems with theirs. I meet with their loved ones, too, sometimes. It is not unusual for me to look directly at the person with hearing loss and ask them a question only to have their loved one answer. I quickly let them know that I am not talking to them and that I'd like the person with the hearing loss to answer me. Sometimes they are taken aback because they are used to answering for them. Yes, it's easier that way. But it devalues the person with the hearing loss. I spoke to an elderly man once and he didn't understand me. So his wife tried to answer again. I didn't let her. Instead, I took his iPad and opened the notebook app and spoke into it. My words appeared on the screen and he read them. He then answered me — in *his* words. He was having a problem with his CI and I needed to know what he was hearing. I also needed him to know my recommendations. But more importantly than that, I needed him to know that what he was going through mattered. It was important to me and to him. It *was* worth my time to communicate with him and to listen to what he had to say. We had a whole conversation after that. His wife was amazed. She hadn't seen him talk like that in quite a while. But I made an effort and so did he.

It's much easier to talk around the person with hearing loss when we are in a group setting. And so they just sit there, excluded. If they have hearing aids, and aren't participating, they likely can't follow the conversation. Bring some pictures to share with them. Use your notepad app to let them know what the conversation is about. Have you heard a funny joke lately? Write it down and show it to them. You don't have to include them in every conversation. That gets exhausting and frustrating for all of you. But let them know that they matter. When you are alone with them again, let them know what the conversations were about. Take the time and whatever you do, don't say, "Never mind"!

If your loved one has recently gotten a cochlear implant, don't put undue expectations on them. Chances are, they are hearing some pretty strange things in the beginning. They will not all of a sudden be able to understand you without reading your lips. That might not happen for many months, if ever, it just depends on their situation. Help them to appreciate the small things to take less pressure off of the big things that might still be frustrating. Did they hear the elevator bell ding? Did they hear the turn signal on the car? Did they hear the chirp of the car being unlocked? Did they hear birds? Did they hear the leaves crunching under their feet? These are insignificant things to people that can hear, but they are incredible things that are all new experiences to the person with a new CI. Celebrate those victories! Help them out with rehab, too. A fun game you can play when you are driving or walking around outside is the "sign game." Read a word that you both can see (don't let them look at you. No lipreading!) and have them repeat it back to you. It will give them confidence. Ask them if there are words that they are having trouble understanding, maybe words beginning with R or L, for example. Then think up words with those letters and see if they can understand them.

Living with hearing loss, quite frankly . . . sucks! It's a lot of hard work. It takes a lot of effort on both the hearing person and the hard of hearing person's behalf. But if you make that effort, you are making a connection. You are giving validation. You are saying, "You're worth it to me." That's really the best gift you can give to anyone.

March 19, 2017 Unpleasant Blast to the Past at the General Hospital Convention

I am a big fan of the soap opera, General Hospital. I admit it. It's my guilty pleasure. I'll let you in on a little secret. I'm actually eight years behind in watching because I don't want to miss an episode. Yep. I actually have eight years of episodes on DVD in my garage.

It was announced that the first annual General Hospital Convention was coming to Burbank. That's about an hour's drive away so, of course, I had to go. Evidently, I'm not *that* big of a fan because I was not willing to pay $550 for the best package with the seats up close, nor $849 to sit in the first row. Those people got to tour the set, which would have been really cool. Instead, I settled for a $60 ticket that got me a reserved seat in row M in the center.

I went with my friend, Lorna, who is also a fan and she is my co-worker, too. The majority of the convention was a couple of celebrity panels where they answered questions. They also showed a recent episode while a couple of the celebrities commented. It was really great to see all of the actors. I knew who the majority of them were and we had great seats.

One of the studio tour groups was late getting back so they had a big delay waiting for them to arrive. They filled the waiting time with two of the actors taking questions from the audience. One of the actors I could understand fairly well. I got maybe 75% of what she said. That was Laura Wright who plays Carly in case you are a fan. Another actor (Griffin) was the one who went around the audience. He had a deep voice and I could not understand a single thing he said. He was loud enough but not clear. Forget about understanding the audience questions. He wasn't holding the microphone in the right place to even pick up those questions. I was a little worried about if I was going to be able to understand the group panels but I held out hope.

As it turns out, I could understand maybe 10% of what was said in the panel discussions. This was, of course, highly disappointing. It actually brought me back to the days when I had my hearing aids and I went to other conventions and could not understand anything there either. I had hoped those days were long gone. Naturally, as was so often the case in my past, I assumed it was just me that couldn't understand anything. Lorna said she was having a hard time, too, but I just thought she was being nice and was trying to make me feel better.

After the panel discussions, most of the people were getting autographs (at $20-$30 each!). Lorna and I went to the vendor area where several of the actors had tables. We were able to chat with several of them (Max, Diane, Lucas, Jordan, and Epiphany). We loved that!

The next day, the General Hospital Facebook page posted videos of a couple of the questions from the panel. I watched, and of course, couldn't understand anything. I read the comments and was quite shocked to learn that *no one* could understand anything. They all complained and said there should have been closed captions. It wasn't just the video that was bad either. It turns out that even the people that paid $550 to sit in the front section couldn't understand anything all day either. Wow! Here I thought I had somehow reverted back to my hard of hearing days and that it was my CI that was the problem, yet it turned out that I was still normal. I was hearing exactly what everybody else was hearing — a really bad sound system that echoed and reverberated.

The good news, for me at least, is that Advanced Bionics has an Echo Block program that helps in situations just like this. Unfortunately for me, I don't have the upgrade yet. If I do get that program before the next convention I will go back. This has definitely given me the incentive to go get it. With the Echo Block advantage, I may be the only one there that understands anything. At least I have hope!

May 15, 2017 I'm Still Amazed

On any given day I pretty much take my good hearing for granted now. But every now and then, I think, "Wow! Can you believe this is happening?" I love to work on jigsaw puzzles. When I do, I turn on the Pandora app on my iPhone and listen to music. On some songs, the lyrics are as clear as if someone is speaking to me in a quiet room. Those are times when I just smile and smile and keep on listening. I really get a kick out of it when I'm listening to one of my favorites like Maroon 5 and that happens. There are a lot of lyrics in some of those songs and it's *really* cool to be able to understand them.

I go to the movies a lot more than I ever used to now. I was using the captioning device. One day I just decided to quit using it cold turkey. The majority of the time, I can actually understand probably 95% of the movie with no problems. I did see *Beauty and the Beast* the other night and I didn't get all of the lyrics in that one but I understood all of the speaking parts. I saw *Born in China* recently. That's the DisneyNature movie that has only one narrator throughout the entire movie and you can't see him. I got every word on that one. I think I will probably get the captioned device for musicals, if there are people with accents, or loud action movies, but for the rest of them, I'll do without. I get a little giddy sometimes sitting there thinking, "Wow! I'm actually getting all of this!"

June 15, 2017 Strange Beeping

I was sitting at my computer at 4:00 am when I kept hearing this annoying beeping sound. What was it, and where was it coming from? I was upstairs and I was actually able to follow the sound. It was coming from downstairs somewhere. It got louder as I went along. First I checked outside. Was it a car alarm? Nope. I stopped and listened again and determined it was coming from the kitchen. I got in there and it was really loud, but what was making the noise? It wasn't the smoke alarm. I listened carefully and continued to follow it. It led me to the microwave which was beeping like crazy. Well, what do you know? It turns out there is a "reminder" button that must have gotten pushed and it was set for 4:12 am. Wow! Who knew?

This occurrence probably would have annoyed most people but I thought it was pretty cool. For starters, I could actually hear the high-pitched beeping all the way upstairs. Secondly, I was able to follow the sound. I could tell where it was coming from and I was able to locate the source pretty quickly. I never would have been able to hear it at all with my hearing aids.

So, why am I awake at 4:00 am? I'm heading to Iceland with my mom tonight and I'm trying to minimize my jet lag when I get there. I'm excited!

June 29, 2017 Blue Lagoon

My mom and I just got back from a trip to Iceland. On our second day, we went to the Blue Lagoon. It was surrounded by lava fields and the color of the water was truly beautiful. It's a geothermal spa and the water is about ninety-nine degrees fahrenheit. In my hearing aid days, I would not have been able to hear anything and if I wanted to have a conversation I would have had to read lips. This time, I put my Neptunes on, clipped them to my bathing suit strap and I was able to listen to everything. I was able to have conversations with my mom, and I definitely heard the Blue Lagoon employee asking me if I wanted to sample the body scrub.

Another *big, big* benefit of cochlear implants is that I could listen to complete silence on the airplane if I chose to. On the flight over to Iceland, I definitely chose to. Not only was there a little kid behind us making a lot of noise but the flight attendants came around after midnight asking if people wanted to buy anything. My poor mom had to listen to it all while trying to sleep but I didn't have to hear a peep, not even the plane engine, which can be quite loud. Ahhh, sometimes it is nice to be able to be completely deaf.

We had a fantastic trip and I was able to understand most of what the tour guide said. I say "most" because he had an accent and, unfortunately, the processor doesn't remove accents. My mom couldn't understand him either sometimes.

August 16, 2017 # My Mom, Margaret "Midge" Husting

My mom is my very best friend. What you may not know is that my mom has had cancer a total of four different times. The first time, the cancer was in her jaw. They had to remove half of her jaw and replace it with a bone from her leg and a titanium plate. The second time, the cancer came on the other side of her face and, while they did not have to remove the jaw, they did have to shave it down and cut some nerves in her face. Needless to say, these surgeries caused her face and lips to be distorted. It also caused a change in her speech. It was no longer as clear as it used to be. Anyone with hearing loss knows how crucial it is for a person to have good lips. In my hearing aid days, if a person didn't have good lips, it was almost pointless to try to talk to them, as I wouldn't be able to understand what they said. I have been extremely grateful that I got my cochlear implants when I did because I have been able to understand my mother's new speech patterns.

We were in Iceland two months ago, as you know from the last chapter. We had a fantastic time. Halfway through that trip, I noticed a new tumor on the outside of her face. We went to her surgeon when we got home and discovered that, this time, it was terminal. Shortly after that, I moved in with her to take care of her. My hearing loss presented some challenges. Because I have been used to complete silence while I sleep, I am not able to wear my cochlear implants. I can't get a good night's sleep because the sounds I hear keep me awake. I awoke often to find my mom sitting up in the bed. I valued these moments, however, because I was able to give her a nice massage and tell her how much I loved her.

I was pretty tired during the daytime, but I had to keep my "ears" on in order to be able to answer the many phone calls that came in and answer the door for all of the visitors and nurses that came to the house. I was so grateful that I was able to understand all of those calls, and hear the doorbell or knocks at the door all of those times. It would have added greatly to my stress level if I didn't have my cochlear implants, as I was often alone with my mother. I enjoyed the many visits that we had. We even did a couple of "FaceTime" visits using my iPhone. It was so gratifying to be able to be able to understand and participate in those visits.

My mother passed away on July 31st. The day before she passed, I had a feeling that time was short. That last night I did wear one of my processors. I lay in the bed next to hers with one ear to the pillow with my eyes closed. The other ear listened to her breathe throughout the night. There were so many different breathing patterns and sounds. I knew she didn't have long. The next morning, I listened to her breathing until at last I realized there was complete silence . . . and she was gone.

We had a heartwarming Celebration of Life party for her last weekend. She didn't want a funeral. She wanted a party. It was a wonderful day with so many friends and family members in attendance. Again, I was grateful for my CIs. I was able to understand everyone that spoke at her service. I could make out the lyrics of the songs that the singer sang. I could understand the prayers that were said while my head was bowed. I could hear all of the kind words that were spoken in my ear while I was embraced in warm hugs by those that cared about me. I could understand all of the funny, loving stories that were told about her at the reception.

My mother is gone now. She was laid to rest on Monday. She will forever be in my heart, though, and I am sure I will continue to hear her lovely voice.

March 12, 2018 # Wild Adventures with Headphones

One of the things I love the most about my Advanced Bionics Naida processor is the AB patented T-Mic. It's a microphone that sits at the base of my ear canal and allows me to use my ears the same way normal hearing people can. For example, I can simply hold any phone up to my ear in the natural position and talk. One of the really great things it allows me to do is wear headphones, just like a normal hearing person can. I'm able to use earbuds, too.

In the past six months I've been on a couple of trips where I got to do some really cool adventures. When I was in Texas, I did the "Future Flight." It looks like a go cart with a giant fan on the back with a big parachute. I have *no* idea how it actually flies, but it does.

I was really excited to find that the headphones and the helmet both fit perfectly. I sat behind the pilot and, thanks to my cochlear implants, I was able to talk to the pilot for the whole hour that we were flying. He pointed out lots of things that we were flying over. He asked me lots of questions and I asked him questions, too. I understood the whole conversation, high up in the air, sitting behind him without being able to see his face.

Last month, I was in New Zealand and Australia for a few weeks with my friend, Tammy. The Sydney BridgeClimb was highly recommended to me by several different people.

It was just as it sounds like. We climbed the Sydney harbor bridge! It took a little over three hours to get to the very top of the bridge and come back down. We went to the very top where the flags are. We were chained to the bridge the whole time so we couldn't change position. The tour guide was in the lead position. I was towards the back of the group. We wore headphones the whole way. The guide told us a lot of stories about the bridge and I was very grateful that I could understand it all. The tour would have been okay in silence, but it was a whole lot better being able to hear the whole time.

June 17, 2018 Hunewill Guest Ranch

Tom and Rama met Steve in church about five years ago. Rama noticed Steve's cochlear implants and she asked him about them. She is hard of hearing. He told her about the Bionic Ear Association socials and they started going a couple of years ago. That's how I met them. I've been Rama's mentor ever since.

Rama and Tom have been going to the Hunewill Guest Ranch in Bridgeport, CA for many years. They invited Steve and I along this year. I went to a horse ranch when I was in the Girl Scouts when I was about twelve. I remember that week, to this day, and it's been on my bucket list for a long time to go to a dude ranch as an adult. I wanted to see if it was as much fun as I remembered it. I jumped at the chance to go to Hunewill.

Rama finally got her cochlear implant. In fact, she was just activated a month ago. She almost canceled the trip because she was concerned that she wasn't going to be able to hear with her new ear. I assured her that she would definitely not hear any worse than she did with two hearing aids and, if anything, it would be much better. Fortunately, she listened and dared to dream.

It is a six and a half hour drive to Hunewill. Rama and Tom drove their own car. Steve doesn't talk much in the car so I suggested that we get an audiobook for us to listen to on the way there and back. I figured it would give him some good rehab to practice listening in the car and it would give me some entertainment along the way. I checked out Dean Koontz' *The City* CDs along with the physical book from the library. I'm pleased to say that I was actually able to understand all but a few words. I was even able to figure out that the narrator was African-American just from listening to him speak. Sure enough, the character in the book was also African-American. I was right. Steve found that he needed to read along to the book in order to fully understand what was said on the CDs. Sometimes he would read a chapter and then listen to it without reading along to help with the rehab. It was a good book that we both enjoyed.

Hunewill was just as great as I had hoped it would be. The scenery was stunning. I fell in love with the horses. Our accommodations were good and the food was great. I rode my horse every morning and afternoon for a couple hours each time. Steve described the rides the best, "Marshland and meadow, rivers and streams, pine needles and bristlecone, valleys and hills, scrub brush and forest — our horses took us through them all!" I got a bit excited when I was able to understand the lady on the horse that was riding behind me on one of the trails. We had a whole conversation with no problem whatsoever. What was even better was that Rama was also able to have conversations while she was riding on her horse. There were two things she really wanted to be able to do: understand the Hispanic wrangler that had an accent and to understand a fellow guest that had a handlebar mustache. She has known both of these men for years and has not been able to read their lips or comprehend what they have been saying. She was finally able to have conversations with both of them, even while riding a horse.

There were a lot of nighttime activities, too. Sadly, Rama has not participated in some of the activities due to her hearing loss. She wasn't going to participate this year, either, but I convinced her to at least give it a try. Steve, Rama and I went to the dance night. We square danced, line danced, and even circle danced. It was great fun. We danced the entire time and I'm pretty sure we each smiled the entire time, too. Each dance had instructions as they were all group dances. All of us were able to follow along with no problem. We could hear the music, too. My feet may need some kind of assisted device, though, because even though I clearly heard "right foot" my left foot moved. Oh well, fortunately, I didn't step on Rama.

They had a campfire and sing-a-long another night. Again, Rama didn't want to go. She just knew she wouldn't be able to hear in the dark and wouldn't know the songs. I told her the same thing I told her on the dance night — just go and if you aren't having a good time, you can leave. They gave us a book with the songs in them. She had no problems following along with what we were singing. I noticed she and Steve were singing, too.

Another night was Talent Night. Rama always loved this activity. She rushed out to save seats in the first row for us so that she would be able to read lips easily. I told her husband that this would be the last year she would be worried about that. He found that hard to believe but I can pretty much guarantee that will not be an issue for her next year. I told horse jokes and Steve showed his calligraphy portfolio. We enjoyed lots of songs, dances, jokes, and more.

One night we drove to a beautiful creek where they had a BBQ dinner set up for us. I had a whole conversation with Rama in the car. She was in the front seat and I was in the back. When we were back at the ranch, I pointed out to her that she was able to have that conversation and she was amazed!

We did some other rehab, too. When we were watching the newborn filly, I told her words that she could see: fence, colt, barn, horse, grass, bird, cow, meadow, etc. She repeated back what she could hear. She didn't get all of the words but she got quite a few.

Our time at the ranch was really a great experience. I got to spend a lot of time with my brother, which I thoroughly enjoyed. We had a lot of laughs together. I got to enjoy nature. I got to watch Rama as she started on her journey. She finally dared to dream and her world is in the process of changing big time!

October 11, 2018 Shark Dive in South Africa

I recently returned from a trip to South Africa. One of the things I was really excited to do was to go on the Shark Dive. Before I left home, I took out my Neptune processor. The Neptune processor is waterproof and would be perfect for the Shark Dive. The last time I used it was over a year ago when I went to Iceland. Unfortunately, I didn't remove the batteries after I last used it. Uh-oh. It turns out there was a bit of corrosion. I tried my best to clean it up but, in doing so, I managed to break a piece of the processor. They are over five-years-old. Valuable lesson learned — remove your batteries when not using your Neptune (or any other electronics for that matter). Fortunately, I have two of them.

The day came for us to go on our dive. I clipped the processor to my bathing suit strap and pulled on the wetsuit. Okay, okay, someone else helped me pull on my wetsuit. Those things are hard to get on! I was very happy to find out that I was able to pull the wetsuit head cover over my headpiece and I could still hear. I could even wear the face mask with no problem.

The cage holds eight people and is attached to the side of the boat. When the shark comes near the cage, they call out "Dive!" and you hold your breath and go under water. There were three groups of us that went into the cage. I was in the third group. The second group got to see several sharks go right up to them and it was pretty exciting. Unfortunately, the sharks didn't come around when I was in the cage. I heard them yell to dive once, but we could not see any sharks. We were in the cage for quite a while hoping the sharks would come back. It was nice to be able to talk to my friend while we were waiting. I definitely would not have been able to do that in the past.

November 14, 2018 # Firsts on a Plane

I just got back from Orlando, Florida. Normally, I like to read books when I travel, especially on planes. This trip was to the Stampin' Up! convention for a few days and the rest of the time was going to be sightseeing. I was going to be with three friends and I knew we weren't going to be getting much sleep. I figured I wouldn't have time to make it through a whole book so I left the books at home. I also got a notification from United Airlines that they would be showing *Mamma Mia: Here We Go Again* on the plane and I really wanted to see that. I knew that people brought their own headphones nowadays, so I searched for some headphones that I bought long ago at the Dollar Store just to see how they would work.

I learned some things when I got on the plane. Some of you may start laughing at me at this point, but when you read physical books on a plane and don't use electronics, you don't know these things. It turns out they have an electrical outlet at each seat now. Who knew? They are on the seat in front of you, pretty low down. That is a great feature. Now I can charge my batteries and my phone on long flights if I need to.

I also discovered that there are no more screens on the seats on the newer planes. On our United Airlines flight, we had to download the United Airlines app onto a mobile device and then watch what we wanted to from the app. Unfortunately, I didn't know that until right before we boarded for the flight to Orlando. The app took forever to load and I had to turn it on airplane mode before it finished. So, no movies for me on that flight. Fortunately, I did bring some magazines to read.

I observed how my friends were watching their movies. I noticed that my older iPhone and iPad had a plug for a headphone jack. My friend's phone is newer and she didn't have that plug on her phone. She did have a converter plug that allowed her to use her headphones with her phone. The bad part was that it used the same plug as the one where the charge cord goes. That meant she could not use her headphones and use the phone charger at the same time. She had to make sure her device was fully charged or she would be out of luck on a long flight. I also found out that we could choose from a lot of movies, not just the newer ones. There were also TV shows and music that we could listen to.

I made sure to load the app onto my iPad and my iPhone before we went back to the airport for our return flight home. One of my friends watched *Mamma Mia* and wasn't too impressed. Another friend watched a "Julie" movie and highly recommended it. I saw another movie offered that I really wanted to see, but had missed when it was in theatres, too. I had my app ready to go and my iPad was fully charged. I plugged in my cheap headphones and tried them out. For dollar headphones, they actually worked. The volume was very low, the airplane noise was very high and I had to hold them close to my T-mics the whole time but . . . they worked! I wasn't able to get the closed captioning to work but I was able to understand the majority of the movies, even with the very poor sound quality. It was a success.

I went to the store to look at headphones but I wasn't able to try them on. I went on the Advanced Bionics Facebook group, and asked what headphones people were using on planes. The most popular answers were to use the ComPilot, Sony headphones that go around the ear (as opposed to over the ear) and Bose Q25 or Q35 headphones. I haven't used my ComPilot in a long time and that option never even crossed my mind. The ComPilot came with my processors. It allows devices like an iPad or iPhone to stream directly to my processors, which makes them act *exactly* like headphones without actually having anything on my ears at all. If I can't connect via Bluetooth on the plane, then I can use a male to male audio cable to plug it in to my device. Fortunately, Advanced Bionics processors have a T-mic, which sits at the opening of the ear canal. It makes wearing headphones very easy.

I will be going to Thailand in January, which will be a very long flight. I'm going to go to Best Buy where I can try out different headphones and see which ones I like the most. I'll bring my books, my ComPilot and maybe some new headphones. I won't stress out about my batteries running out of charge either.

December 13, 2018 Triumph Over My Greatest Fear

For fifty-two years I've been terrified of bugs! I know what you are thinking, "Seriously? You have: gotten in a cage to see sharks, pet a cheetah and lions, skydived, ziplined, gone whitewater rafting, driven a formula Ford on a race track, and you're terrified of . . . crickets?!" Yes, it's true. I only killed bugs if I had bug spray and even then I would never pick them up to throw them away. If a bug was in my house, I would put a cup over it and wait for Bob to kill it when he got home. I was extremely afraid of crickets and cockroaches, but definitely didn't care for spiders or any other bugs either.

My friends have had some good laughs over my fears. Just mention the words "Julie" and "Japanese beetles" to my friend, Marsha, and watch her go into hysterics. Other friends have *not* been pleased with my fear. Just ask my friend, Tammy, about being woken out of a pleasant sleep in order to kill a bug in the hotel room.

It was in January of this year that Tammy and I were in Uluru, Australia, near Ayer's Rock. Uluru is in the middle of nowhere. It's the perfect place to see stars in all of their glory. It's also heaven for, you guessed it. Bugs! Tammy and I took a bus tour to what was supposed to be a lavish dinner under the evening stars. A lecturer was to show us the various stars and it was to be an exquisite sight to see. I should have realized when there were too many clouds to see any stars that we were headed for disaster. There were large round tables with lights in the center of the tables. Those were the only lights around. In case you didn't know, bugs flock to lights. Since those were the only lights around, the bugs were jumping and crawling and flying onto our table all night long. All kinds of bugs. I will not go into detail, as some of you may also share my fear and I don't want to give you nightmares. Needless to say, I didn't eat much of my dinner and I skipped dessert. If you know me, you know it's a big deal for me to skip dessert. Since it was a bus tour, I couldn't just get up and leave either. I endured that personal hell for about three hours. Tammy got a bit angry at my hysterics and, honestly, I can't blame her.

It was my first trip with Tammy and I knew I had to take care of this irrational fear once and for all if I ever hoped to travel with her or anyone else again. I had always wanted to try hypnosis to get over my fear. Unfortunately, hypnotherapy requires you to close your eyes and be in a very calm state. It requires listening carefully with your eyes closed. That was impossible for me to do when I had hearing aids. But now I have cochlear implants. Would it finally be possible to try this approach? The worst that could happen if it didn't work is I would be out $150 and two hours of my life. I decided to give it a try.

A friend gave me a recommendation, I made the appointment and off I went. It turns out that the fears people have of being hypnotized — you lose all control, you don't know what they are doing to you, they make you do painful things — are all false. I knew exactly what she told me. I did have to give her examples of the times I was the most terrified and that did get me very upset and made me cry. She needed to see my reaction before we started. She asked me to tell her these same stories when we were finished so she could see how much my reaction had changed. It was very easy to relate those stories at the end of our session. I was pretty skeptical when I left because I didn't feel any differently. I also never felt like I was really hypnotized because I *was* in control and I *did* know and remember everything she said.

It wasn't too long after my appointment that a silverfish showed up in my house. Poor guy never stood a chance! I even used a Kleenex to kill it. I was pretty proud of myself but still was a bit skeptical. Silverfish seemed pretty easy. One day, Bob saw a big spider in the kitchen and told me to stay away and asked where the bug spray was. I walked in and said, "Oh, let me get that for you." I swatted it and threw it away. Wow! Maybe this really *did* work. A couple months later a dying cricket came into the house. I didn't know it was dying at the time. I killed it and threw it away. A full on live cricket came another time. Yep! I got him! I just got back from Orlando, and there were tiny roaches in our condo there. They didn't bother me. I was able to sleep knowing that they were around. There was even one on my chair and I casually got up and moved away. My friends that knew of my fear were amazed. So was I, to tell you the truth.

If you have a fear of heights, bugs, or flying, or you need to stop smoking or lose weight, or anything else you can't conquer on your own, I *highly* recommend a session with a hypnotherapist. It was the best $150 and two hours I ever spent. I'm *so* grateful for my cochlear implants so that I could finally conquer my greatest fear. I'm going to Thailand and Cambodia with Tammy in January and I have a feeling she will be grateful as well.

March 1, 2019 Even the Littlest Things Make My Day!

I purchased a new printer yesterday. It's an Epson ET-2750. I chose it because I was tired of paying so much for ink cartridges. This printer is different. It has "tanks" in the printer that hold the ink instead of using cartridges. The ink comes in bottles and you pour it into the tanks. The ink is designed to automatically stop coming out of the bottle when it reaches the fill line. I followed the instructions and, to my surprise, I heard the gurgle, gurgle, gurgle of the ink going into the tank. Once you fill it up, you have to follow some other instructions and then you have to top it off. When I went to put the ink in the second time, I heard the gurgle for the first color but didn't hear it for the second color. I knew that I needed to take it off and put it back on and, sure enough, there was the gurgle.

I got the biggest kick out of that glug, glug, glug sound. Ha! I definitely would not have been able to hear that with my hearing aids. I would have had to really pay attention to the fill lines and I have a feeling that second color would not have gotten topped off if I had to look to see if it happened. I filled the whole thing just by listening to a faint sound. Wow!

May 9, 2019 R/C Cars

My dad was one of the original pioneers in the R/C (radio-controlled) car industry. His name is Gene Husting and he was co-owner of Associated Electrics aka Team Associated. My brother, Curtis, and I used to race on road cars forty years ago. Curtis has started racing again and he asked me if I wanted to play. I forgot how much fun it is. I've gone to the track about four times now just to practice. I need a *lot* of practice. Ha!

Curtis says I'm not good enough to actually race yet, but he does. I watched him during the qualifying round last night. My "wow" moment came when I was able to clearly understand the announcer over the loud speaker. He told what was going to happen that night. The qualifying rounds have a staggered start. He called out each driver's name, one at a time, for them to begin. Then he announced how they were doing during the round. When I raced back in the day, my mom was known as "Killer" (she raced, too) and I was "Killer Jr." When I do get to finally compete it will be cool to hear the announcer call out my name.

June 3, 2019 *Menopause – The Musical!*

Before I was activated with my first cochlear implant, I made up a wish list of everything I hoped to be able to do once I had it. There were thirteen items on the list. Two of them have been hit or miss–understanding the characters on the rides at Disney parks and understanding plays and musicals. Yesterday, I went to see *Menopause – The Musical.*

It was playing at the Welk Theatre in Escondido, CA. The theater is small with only about three hundred seats. Every seat is a good seat and the acoustics were very good. Since it was a musical, there was very little talking. It was almost all singing. The songs were taken from the melodies of very popular songs. They just changed the words.

I went to my seat (row F on the end), changed to my music program (80 IDR with no ClearVoice) and crossed my fingers. A woman came out and stood on the floor in front of the stage and talked for a little bit before the show started. She was quite funny, and I understood her perfectly. Then the show began. They talked for a little bit, and I understood them with no problem. Then they started singing. It was great! I was able to make out probably 80% – 100% of the words to the songs, depending on who was singing. It helped that I was able to clearly see their faces. The melodies were all from songs that I was familiar with and I recognized almost all of them. I thoroughly enjoyed the show. I got laughing so hard I cried on one of the songs. If you are going through, or have been through menopause, or you live with someone that has, I highly recommend it. It was a great experience and I was especially happy with the small venue.

You may be wondering what else was on my wish list. These are the items I have been able to cross off — some took longer than others:

- Enjoying concerts
- Understanding conversations while rubber stamping (crafting) with my friends
- Understanding conversations in restaurants
- Understanding people speaking at meetings
- Hearing birds
- Hearing bikes coming up behind me while hiking on trails
- Understanding conversations in the dark
- Understanding conversations in the car
- Understanding dialogue at the movies
- Getting rid of my horrendous tinnitus
- Being able to hear my cat (her meow was my favorite sound)
- Understanding on the phone without assistance

Afterword

As you may have guessed, my story will never end. It's been over six years since I got my first cochlear implant and I'm still amazed at what I am able to do. It is easy to take my good hearing for granted. As a mentor, however, I'm reminded often of what my life used to be like. I meet people regularly that are just beginning this journey.

When I started this journey, I simply hoped to be able to hear well some day. I didn't know how much my life was going to change. I'm grateful to be able to give back as a mentor. I also enjoy being the Orange County, California Chapter Leader for Advanced Bionics' Bionic Ear Association (BEA). When I was younger, I had always thought it would be neat to be an inspirational speaker. Now that dream is fulfilled as I get to do presentations at our BEA socials and sometimes I'm asked to speak at other places as well. I have included two of the presentations I have given in the Appendix on the following pages. I have placed them there for you to easily refer to them in the future and, if you are beginning this journey, I hope you will reread them at the various stages you encounter. I think that they will help you.

I have also included my surgery tips and activations tips in the Appendix as a reference. I suggest reading them, again, a week or two before your surgery and activation dates.

I hope you will visit my blog, too, for my continuing story that goes beyond the contents of this book. Go to: juliehusting.wordpress.com If you need mentoring and/or have any questions or comments, you can write to me at: JulieHusting@gmail.com.

Thank you for going on this journey with me!

161

Appendix

Success Comes When Expectations are Realistic

A lady that was thinking about getting a cochlear implant (CI) did a lot of research. She also went to a lot of meetings about cochlear implants. She qualified for one, and was definitely reading lips and struggled with what she was hearing on a daily basis. She was pretty much convinced that it was time for her to get a cochlear implant, but then she went to a meeting where there were some people with CIs. There was a captioned presentation and she noticed that some of the people with CIs were reading the captions. She determined that they weren't doing any better than she was with her hearing aids so she shouldn't get a CI. She decided they weren't a success.

In order to be successful with a CI, it is crucial that you understand the process that you have to go through. Getting a cochlear implant is not the same thing as getting a hearing aid or glasses. You don't put it on and all of a sudden you hear perfectly. Imagine a scale that runs from one to ten with one being completely deaf and ten being perfect hearing. It is unlikely that a person with a CI is ever going to get to ten. In fact, it can take years to get to an eight if you get there at all. The key to "success" requires having realistic expectations. You need to appreciate every move along the scale on your way to the top. If you don't recognize the little gains along the way, it will be a very disappointing experience.

What can you expect? Before you begin the journey, you are likely a one or two on the scale. You think you are doing just fine with your hearing aids, but in fact, you have to read lips pretty much 100% of the time. Even then, you are missing many of the words. You use facial cues a great deal and you probably use the ol' "smile and nod" on a daily basis because, let's face it, sometimes it's just easier. You're exhausted at the end of the day from concentrating so much. Hearing aids make words louder, but they don't make words clear. It's like holding a microphone up but you are still hearing using a damaged ear.

A cochlear implant bypasses the damaged areas and goes directly to the auditory nerve. Words can then become clear. The brain, however, is a bit confused in the beginning. It's never heard using this kind of technology before and it has to learn how to use it. If you got a knee replacement, you wouldn't be walking well right out of surgery. Your brain has to figure out how to use that new knee. You go home with a walker. You do a lot of rehab exercises. You move up to using a cane. You exercise some more. You ditch the cane and walk with a limp. You exercise some more. Finally, you can walk well again with no pain. You have to teach your brain how to use the new ear just like you would have had to teach it how to use the new knee. Unfortunately, with an ear you can't physically see and feel the changes as the brain progresses like you can with a knee. But you *can* hear the differences along the way.

You *will* hear new things on the very day of your activation. That is the day that the cochlear implant is turned on. What you will hear depends on a lot of different factors: your age, how long you've had bad hearing, how long you had good hearing, how long you kept your auditory nerve stimulated with a hearing aid, etc. I can pretty much guarantee you that you will not hear voices the way you are used to hearing them on day one. You may hear very deep Darth Vader voices or perhaps you will hear high pitched voices like the munchkins in *The Wizard of Oz*. You may even hear R2D2 from *Star Wars* where you hear beeps for speech. Or maybe you will hear the "wah-wah-wah" of Charlie Brown's teacher. It sounds like it would be horrifying but it's really not. Even with those sounds, with lip reading, you can still communicate.

The appreciation part comes in when you realize all of the new sounds that you will hear. You will likely hear steps on the floor, paper shuffling, elevator bells dinging, car turn signals, the beep or click when the car door is unlocked, traffic outside, your car tires on the asphalt, etc. These are all sounds that you probably haven't heard in a long time. You might even be able to play the sign game. If you try to understand without reading lips you won't be able to. But, if you look at a sign and someone reads one of the words that are on the sign, you may be able to pick out the word that was said without reading their lips. This is great rehab when you are in the car (not while you are the driver) or are out walking around.

When you are first activated, your hearing range is at the very bottom of your audiogram. A normal person's hearing is towards the top. Your brain will begin craving more and more volume. You will be sent home with programs that will allow you to add more and more volume to keep up with your brain. Eventually, you will reach the volume level of a normal hearing person. As you climb higher in volume, the strange voices that you heard on the first day will become a bit more normal. My brother, Steve, first said I sounded like R2D2 (beeps for speech) when he was activated. I then turned into C3PO (robotic speech) and now I'm Princess Leia (human speech). One thing that happens during this process is that you will realize how loud you are speaking in relation to everyone else. If you talk too loud (as you likely did when you wore hearing aids) you will hurt your ears so you will automatically start talking softer. You may not appreciate that change, but your friends and relatives definitely will.

If you do rehab exercises, you will begin to hear the differences in words like sin, thin, tin, bin, win, etc. As these words become clearer to you, you will likely begin speaking more clearly yourself. Many people with hearing loss have a "deaf accent" because they can't hear those words clearly. With a CI, you can and you will hear yourself saying the words incorrectly. Eventually, you just start speaking more clearly. You likely may not even realize it, but your friends and family will notice the difference.

Those are the things you can expect in the beginning. Will you still have to read lips? Yes. Will you be able to use the phone? Probably not. Will you be able to enjoy music? Most likely not. The first, and most important goal, is to understand speech clearly. Once you can do that, the rest of it is icing on the cake. That is where realistic expectations come into play. If your definition of success means that you are only successful if you can go to a play and understand every word then you will likely be highly disappointed. If your idea of success means that you can have a conversation without having to work so hard at understanding the words (even though you may still have to read lips) and that you won't come home exhausted, you will be successful. It's best to just enjoy each phase as it comes rather than setting unrealistic goals.

As time goes by, you will begin to move up the scale. Read the next chapter called "How Long Does it Take?" to get an idea of how much time it takes. When you get to full volume and words become clearer, you will find that you don't have to sit in the front row anymore. You may still need to read captions or lips at presentations, but it won't take as much effort. You will no longer have the anxiety of "what if I don't get the best seat?" Again, take the time to appreciate this new phase.

Eventually, you'll get to the point where you won't need to read lips as much. Unfortunately, this change happens very slowly and you may not even realize that you aren't reading lips. I have had many people say they are still reading lips. Then I test them and they understand me just fine without reading my lips. This happens when you least expect it. I didn't know I wasn't reading lips anymore until the person I was speaking to turned their head and I realized I was still understanding her. During this phase, you will be able to enjoy conversations at meals easier. You will be able to have conversations in the car easier. You may even be able to have a conversation with someone in another room. If you look down, or someone turns their head while speaking, you can still follow along in the conversation. You may be able to understand in the dark.

Once you get to that stage, the next triumph is being able to hear on the phone. You can do rehab for listening on the phone. Just like the sign game that I mentioned earlier, you can have someone call you and have them read words to you from a list or book that you can read along with. If you just try to listen, you likely won't understand them. But if you can read along to what they are saying, your brain will make the connection, and you may be able to understand the words. Eventually, you will be able to have regular conversations.

Music and phone use are a bit further up the scale. In the beginning, all music is going to sound like screeching cats. It's going to sound horrible. Don't try to listen to any music that you aren't very familiar with in the beginning. If you do listen to music that you are familiar with, don't be surprised if it sounds like someone else is singing the songs. You may not even be able to tell if it's a woman or a man singing. You may want to listen to instrumental music in the beginning. Some people find piano music to be the best in the beginning. For rehab, I recommend listening to one song that you know well every few days. You will then be able to hear the changes that your ear is going through. The song should not be a "busy" song — i.e., not a lot of instruments or background vocals. Eventually, music will sound better and better to you but it can take a long time before it does.

Some environments are going to be hard for you even when you get near the top of the scale. Fortunately, there are programs and accessories to help you in noisy situations, or out in the wind, or in places that echo, for example. Hard floors and high ceilings are not your friend. If you need assistance in those situations, you are not a failure!

I highly recommend that you keep a hearing journal to chart your progress. Write down the date, new sounds that you are hearing and things that you are still struggling with. In the beginning, you are going to hear new things every day and changes happen very quickly as you move up the volume range. Eventually, all of those "wow" moments are going to become fewer and farther between . . . but they will happen! You may become frustrated and feel like you are stuck in place. That is where the journal comes in. When you feel that frustration you should read your journal. You will have a physical record of all of the things that you can do that you couldn't do with hearing aids. You will also see things that you had a hard time with in the beginning that may be easy later. It's nice to actually be able to *see* your ears move from the walker to the cane to walking on its own. The journal helps you to physically see the progress you are making.

Remember the lady in the beginning that thought the CI people were no better off than she was because they were reading the captions? There could have been so many different reasons why they were using the captions. Maybe the acoustics in the room made it hard to hear. Maybe they were newly implanted and hadn't gotten to the point where they could go without reading lips easily. Maybe they didn't need to read the captions but didn't realize it. Maybe the person didn't speak clearly. In any event, the volume was likely good, and they likely could sit anywhere they wanted. They also probably heard the words clearly and weren't struggling to understand.

It turns out that the woman *did* get a cochlear implant. She is still low on the scale, as she is new, but she has heard things she hasn't heard in years! She even had a conversation with some people that she could never understand before because their lips were too hard to read.

The key is to set your expectations low so that you won't be disappointed. Don't expect to go from zero to ten overnight. Appreciate all of the little gains that you make along the way. In the grand scheme of things, a year of changes is just a blip in the rest of your life! Always remember the three P's — practice, patience and persistence. Enjoy the journey!

How Long Does It Take?

The number one question that I am asked is, "How long did it take you to understand speech with your CI alone?" I normally will not answer that question . . . until now. The answer is . . . four hundred hours of listening to sound with only my processor on and no hearing aid in the other ear. That is when I first noticed. It was 880 hours when I realized I could do it well. If you noticed, I didn't say "one month" or "two months". That is because the brain has to be forced to use the CI, otherwise, it will use whatever is easiest. In order to force the brain to use the CI, you have to remove your hearing aid or plug up your good ear. I did not wear a hearing aid at all after I was activated. I wore my CI, by itself, for sixteen hours a day and I slept for the other eight, so that part doesn't count. Let me give you some things to think about.

Are you right-handed, left-handed, or ambidextrous (use both hands equally well)? Only about 1% of the population is ambidextrous. When we are very young we are trained how to write. Typically, people are trained using their right hand. They write the letters over and over and over again until they get it right. The brain then figures out that "Oh! It's easier to use my right hand so I will continue using it." Does that mean that you can't write with your left hand? No. Does that mean that your "bad" hand (in this case, your left hand) can't do other things? No. If you have learned how to use a computer keyboard properly, then you type equally well with both of your hands. If you are a musician and play the piano or flute, for example, you play your instrument using both hands equally well. But, if you are right-handed, you likely use your right hand to brush your teeth, brush your hair, feed yourself, and do most other tasks throughout the day. So, what would you do if you broke your fingers in your right hand and had to have a cast over your whole hand? Would you starve to death? Would you have someone else feed you for the whole time you have your cast? Of course not! You would train your left hand to do the job that your right hand used to do. And, because your right hand was in a cast, you would be forcing your brain to do it. Would it be awkward at first? Of course! Would it be difficult? Of course! Would it be frustrating? Of course! Would you likely poke your face with a fork a few times or spill food in your lap before finally getting good at feeding yourself? Of course! But eventually, your brain would figure it out and adapt and it would use your "bad" left hand just as well as it did your "good" right hand.

Now let's pretend you and your friend, Jay, wanted to learn Japanese. You both sign up for the same one hour online class. You stay in America, take the class at the same time each day and don't do anything else in Japanese the other twenty-three hours of your day. Jay decides he really wants to learn it quickly. He moves to a remote village in Japan where he lives with a Japanese family. The whole village speaks only Japanese and so does the family he lives with. The signs are also in Japanese. When he goes to a restaurant or to the store, all he hears is Japanese being spoken around him. He takes the same one hour course that you do. But he is hearing the words that he has learned in his lessons throughout the day. He is also hearing many other words that don't make sense to him. But he's listening, and picking up the dialect, the rhythm of the words, and he is trying to use the words that he has learned in each lesson. Who do you think will pick up Japanese the fastest and who will actually remember it when your class is finished — you or Jay?

By removing my hearing aid, I forced my brain to use my cochlear implant. I didn't give it a choice. I did one hour of "active" rehab every night. I listened and read along to audiobooks for thirty minutes every day and I did thirty minutes of various apps and other programs. For the other fifteen hours a day, I listened to music. I talked to people. I went for walks outside to hear other sounds. I went to restaurants. I watched TV. I went to movies. If I had only done that one hour of rehab and then put my hearing aid back in, it would be like taking the class without doing any homework or using the skills that I was learning.

If you have been doing the rehab every day for an hour for two months but put your hearing aid back on the rest of the time, then consider that you have put in sixty hours. At that rate, you probably have about another year to go before you begin to understand without reading lips — assuming you keep practicing diligently for that year. Now maybe you've had your CI for years and think it's too late for you. It's not. I was activated about the same time as a friend of mine. It's been over five years. She refused to take her hearing aid out. For five years, she insisted her hearing aid was better. Her audiologist recently gave her a challenge. She was asked to keep her hearing aid off for thirty days. She has done it and has heard things in that thirty days that she hadn't heard in five years! She just finished her challenge. Now she is going to keep going with it because she can see how beneficial it has been for her.

I can't promise you that you will not need to read lips if you go for a month or two without wearing your hearing aid. There are other factors that play a role in how fast we get to that point. Some of it has to do with age, how long you had good hearing before you began losing your hearing, how long your auditory nerve was stimulated, etc. But I will promise you that in the majority of cases, you will be much better off than you are now. Will it be awkward? Yes! Will you be frustrated? Yes! Will you want to give up? Yes! Will it be worth it in the long run? *Yes*! So, quit making excuses and just do it! I challenge you!

CI Tips — Surgery

Here are some surgery tips for you. Keep in mind that everybody is different so some of these things may, or may not, happen to you. For a couple of weeks after my first surgery, my mouth would not open very wide so I couldn't eat things like hamburgers, for example. Sometimes people have sore jaws for a short time. You might want to stock up on soft foods just in case.

Some people get dizzy and/or nauseous. My surgeon had me wear a prescription seasick patch the night before the surgery. I took it off a couple days afterwards so I never had any of those symptoms. But it's a good idea to be prepared for it. Maybe keep some 7-Up and crackers on hand, and even a bag in the car for the ride home. You might not feel like eating. If that's the case, you might want to have some clear soup on hand. You will likely be told not to bend over for a while and you won't be allowed to lift anything over ten pounds I think it is. It's a good idea not to make any sudden movements, too.

Some people are uncomfortable sleeping in their bed the first night or two. It helps to keep your head elevated. I slept on my recliner for the first few nights. Some people get a travel pillow like you would use on a plane, for their bed.

Be prepared to rest, nap, and get more rest. Your body is going to be really tired and it won't be unusual for you to get very sleepy. Be sure to allow yourself time to heal, and listen to your body. It's not unusual for this to go on for a week.

Sneezing can be painful. Here's a goofy tip but it really works. To stop a sneeze do this: as soon as you get that tickle that indicates you are going to sneeze, flick your tongue back and forth on the roof of your mouth. Start practicing now. If you do it too late you won't be able to stop it in time. If that happens, do a full blown sneeze with your mouth open. Don't try to stop it.

You will hear strange sounds between your surgery and activation. Don't worry about that. It's completely normal. I heard a lot of weird creaking noises. I liked to imagine that my ear was waking up after a long nap.

Occasionally I would hear really loud blasts like a horn honking, but fortunately, those were very short and didn't happen very often.

You may have some loss of taste. Go and eat your favorite foods between now and your surgery. Live it up! I had a slight change in taste after the first surgery, and more after the second. It's kind of like a metallic taste in my mouth. Some foods like bread were very dry and I'd get thirsty but it's not that bad. I could still taste chocolate. Your mouth feels very dry. It's almost like when you feel like you need to brush your teeth when you wake up. These are not supposed to be permanent side effects, by the way, so don't worry too much if this happens to you.

I had been told by many people that the third day was the worst day so I kept expecting the worst but it never came. I was lucky that I didn't have to take any pain medication either. I took a Tylenol now and then before I went to bed but that was it. I could eat easily with no jaw problems after my second surgery, too.

I hope I'm not scaring you. I just want you to be prepared for the possibility of any of these things happening and to know that if any of them *do* happen, you shouldn't panic.

You will need to wear a button down or zippered shirt when you go in for surgery. You will wake up with a goofy cone over your ear and you won't be able to pull a regular shirt over your head.

Have you started your wish list yet? It's time to start walking around as a hearing person would. Look around you and make a list of the things you hope to hear/understand some day. It's fun to check them off!

CI Tips – Activation

Your activation is coming soon! Here are some tips to help you prepare for your big day and the days afterwards. Keep one thing in mind. Your activation day is going to be the best day and worst day of your whole journey. It will be the best day because your cochlear implant will finally be turned on. That will bring relief that it works and excitement for what's to come. However, it also happens to be the very worst day of what you are going to be hearing. Remember that your ear hasn't heard this way in a long time, if ever, and the brain needs to relearn how to hear using this new method. So what you hear when you are activated is like a newborn baby coming out. It has a lot to learn.

It's a good idea to hope for the best but expect the worst so that you won't be disappointed. It is not unusual *not* to understand speech when you are activated. You may hear beeps or tones or even "waa waa waa" when people are talking to you, like Charlie Brown's teacher. That is completely normal. My brother told me I sounded like R2D2 (beeps for speech) from *Star Wars* when he was first activated. A few days later I turned into C3P0 (robot). A couple of months later I was Princess Leia (human), so it does get better.

You will need to do rehab exercises to train your brain to listen with the CI. I highly recommend getting audiobooks and the physical book so that you can read along with it while you listen. You can get both from the library. You may need to start with children's books and work your way up to novels. If you try to listen to the audio without reading along, you likely will not understand it. However, when you read along, your brain will soon pick up the speech.

I also recommend that you use this time before activation to make up a list of "closed set" words. Closed set words are when you have a category and a list of words that go in that category. For example, the category might be "days of the week" and the words would be Wednesday, Friday, etc. Mix up the words. Months, holidays, family names, numbers, and favorite TV shows or other things that you like (flowers, animals, etc.) are good closed set words. Have someone tell you the category so that you understand what the category is, and then have them read the words in random order without you looking at them (close your eyes or have them stand near your ear but where you can't see them). Even if you are only hearing beeps, you might be surprised that you can actually get the words right. The brain is an awe-inspiring thing!

Another fun game to play is what I call the sign game. When you are in the car with someone, have them pick out words from signs that you can both easily see — choose only signs on the right side of the road, for example. You won't understand what they say but you may very easily pick out the word on a sign. This also works during the "beeping" stage. You can even do this on the way home from your activation. It may surprise you.

I have a Facebook daily rehab group where I post four exercises each day: an audio exercise, an Angel Sound program exercise, a phone exercise and an "extra credit" exercise which adds some variety. Search for "Cochlear Implant Daily Rehab" on Facebook to find and join the group. I highly recommend an hour of rehab a day using only your CI ear. Do not use a hearing aid with it. It's important that you give your new ear stimulation. If you are used to a quiet house, turn the TV or radio on just to have something for your ear to listen to. The more you can go without your hearing aid, the better.

You are about to embark on an amazing journey! Get ready to cross items off of your wish list!

Acknowledgements

I have some people to thank that were valuable to me at different stages of this journey:

My friend, Bob Jones – when you first met me at work you thought I was a stuck up snob that was ignoring you because I didn't acknowledge you when you spoke to me. You have shown great patience to me over the years and you have repeated yourself so many times without complaining!

My brother, Steve, for going on this journey with me. You are the one person that has understood my difficulties, firsthand, and it was a great relief to know I wasn't going to be alone in this process. I appreciate your helping me turn this book from a dream into a reality, too.

My brother, Curtis, and my parents for always giving me support.

Wendy Meyer-Eberhard, the audiologist who first suggested that I get a cochlear implant. Who knows how long it would have taken if you hadn't made the suggestion?

Al and Debbie Vantwist — Al is the first person I met that had a cochlear implant. The one hour that Steve, Shirley and I met with you changed our fear to excitement for which I will always be grateful. You are also the reason that I became a mentor. I wanted to do for others what you did for me.

Lori Shapiro, the friend that put this all in motion by suggesting I start a blog.

Dr. Jack Shohet, my kind, compassionate and very skilled surgeon that performed this miracle.

Cheryl Tanita, my first audiologist that was willing to do whatever I asked.

Sarah Hargest, the Advanced Bionics employee that convinced me to become the Orange County BEA Chapter Leader.

The Original Ci Breakfast Club — they were the tiny rehab group I joined when I first started. You supported me day in and day out and have become very good friends. You also inspired me to start my Facebook rehab group, that has since helped thousands of people.

The Advanced Bionics research team — for letting me give back by being a tiny part of your incredible work and for all you do to make our lives better.

My fellow mentors — you help, inspire, encourage, and make so many lives better every day. I'd especially like to thank David Ryan for being a great mentor to me, personally.

The people that I have mentored — there are too many to name but I so appreciate your letting me be a part of your journey. It is very rewarding to get to see where you started to where you are now. It fills my heart to get to be lucky enough to be a part of your lives.

Alison Eier, the Advanced Bionics representative that I currently work with. You are so good at what you do and I'm privileged to get to work with you.

Deb Boone — thank you for helping me edit this book.

My friends — there are too many to name but you know who you are. You've been there for me in good times and bad. You've undoubtedly repeated yourself many times for which I am grateful! You've seen my laughter and tears and have been a part of it all.